Slam The Door On Cancer

And Lock It Out of Your Life

By Jacquie Woodward

Unless otherwise noted, Scripture quotations taken from the Amplified® Bible. Copyright 1954,
1958, 1962, 1964, 1965, 1987 by The Lockman Foundation. Used by permission.
(www.Lockman.org)

All Bible references taken from WordSearch Bible Software, Austin, TX. USA.
www.wordsearchbible.com , unless otherwise noted.

All boldface in Scripture references are added by author of this book for emphasis.

The use of lower case "s" in the word satan is intentional as a refusal to honor that name.

Disclaimer: This book is neither intended to provide medical advice nor replace professional
health care consultation. The author has no business connection with any product mentioned.

Light Heir Media, LLC
PO Box 719
Burgin, KY 40310

www.slamthedooroncancer.com
(email "contact" link provided on this website)

Dedication:

This book is a gift to my children and their children with my prayer for them to live in the "healthy state" and to my husband who has honored me by embracing living in the healthy state with me.

It is also a memorial to my mother, Evelyn Grace Wash who donated her body to scientific research upon her death at age 93 never truly receiving the commemoration she richly deserved. She gracefully lived the pure laws of health—love, work, and stewardship.

Acknowledgements:

My sincere gratitude to:

Father God for almost daily "downloads" and the opportunity to be an encourager.

My family for loving me through the "valley of the shadow of death" every step of the way.

Blue Moth Media and Julia Loren for putting me on track and keeping me there with amazing wisdom and skill. (www.bluemothmedia.com)

Kelly Laymon of Laymon Designs for sensitive and skillful work on the blog for this book: www.slamthedooroncancer.com

Harold Delk, Lynelle Cain, and Carol Ann Tramontin for being obedient "earthly angels".

My physicians and caregivers who made tremendous efforts in the midst of extraordinarily difficult circumstances.

April Tyler, Jill Cutler, Bob and Kaye Jobe, Pastor Pam Sims, Pastor Geoff Barrett, Aprile Hunt, Diana Draper, Donna Conder, Pastor Tom Lane, Carlene Wheeler, Pat McDaniel, and all who patiently read manuscripts and gave me honest feedback and encouragement. Pete Presley, Kris Watts, and Lora Konstantinova for their artistic contributions.

Table of Contents

Foreword

I am excited about Jacquie Woodward's book and testimony!

This is the extraordinary true story of her reality for you or any believer to "Slam The Door On Cancer ... And Lock It Out Of Your Life"

The book reads not like eloquent and lucid presentations of complex ideas regarding the disease, cancer, or like an advanced understanding of science including quantum physics. Rather it simply tells her story as if it was a series of adventures--adventures in revelation, in God's Word, and in opening her portal for healing and the power and authority of Jesus's name.

Her writing tells her stories with enthusiasm and explains physics with clarity. Her "Sources and References Appendix " is a remarkable resource for powerful reading.

Here is her story of moving from:

- ❖ sickness to hope. .
- ❖ disease to health
- ❖ having little insight to powerful revelation.

It is an open portal of God's Word from death unto abundant life!

May this awesome book find it's way to many cancer victims. May the more than 60 printed Scriptures in the "Appendix One" bring readers to the deliverance that Jacquie Woodward has found.

David Van Koevering
Elsewhen Research
www.elsewhen.com

About the Author

Who would write a book entitled, *Slam the Door on Cancer...and Lock It Out of Your Life*? The answer is someone who, perhaps like you, was shocked to hear the dreaded "C Word" pronounced over her life sending her reeling and wondering who sucked all the air out of the room.

The answer is a wife, mother, and grandmother who was not finished creating a legacy. The answer is a long dormant Christian who suddenly realized she wanted to bear more fruit before leaving this earth.

The answer is a woman who found herself with two strikes against her and only one choice - hit a home run. And, because her "batting coach" gave her perfect signals, she did.

Jacquie Woodward lives in Kentucky with her husband. She is available to speak and bring her encouraging message to your venue. You may see more about her book, find her inspirational blog and many resources to help motivate you towards living in a state of health on her website at:

www.slamthedooroncancer.com

To invite Jacquie to speak to your group contact her via the email contact link on this website:

Introduction

"It's cancer!" Too shocking and too common! When I heard, "You have a mass in your pancreas," I desperately needed the book I offer here because highly specialized "medical science" had little to offer me except, perhaps, risky surgery. Available literature seemed as compartmentalized as orthodox medicine emphasizing either diet, alternative cures, or mind-body theories. I needed the truth regarding each of those focuses efficiently delivered because time was of the essence.

I also needed a greater truth I didn't realize right away. I'll share throughout this book how that truth found me and pulled all the facets of healing together in an "interactive miracle" which is really the seminal insight I must share herein.

Early on, a physician friend told me candidly, "If you want to live through this, you will have to be your own doctor." Then she quipped, "I think I read somewhere that you should eat a lot of blueberries." Turns out her advice was some of the most helpful I received. Although I don't intend for this book to be about me, I will share my story to illustrate and to encourage.

My husband, a , pediatrician spent the second half of his career in care management witnessing at close range the results of orthodox cancer treatment protocols. Over the years I had been privy to enough doctor conversations to form a great many questions about cancer diagnosis and treatment and I share some of these in this book. Nevertheless, leaving the familiar is difficult. It would have amounted to heresy for me to consider an "alternative cancer treatment" even though we knew the limitations of orthodox protocols. I also knew my husband would struggle with my pursuing anything not scientifically substantiated.

As I researched, several alternative cure regimens were attractive because they work with the body's innate healing mechanisms - a principle I have employed in my own healing. I soon realized the futility of expecting that any expert, whether considered orthodox or alternative, would be the sole agent to snatch me from cancer's grasp.

I eventually realized that "I" was not my body; and if "I" wanted a healthy body in which to live out my natural lifespan, "I" would have to FULLY participate in the healing of that body. That participation included dealing with the cause of the cancer attack. Walk with me through my interactive miracle where "I", a long dormant Christian, learned to tune into my Creator to hear how He wanted to manifest my healing, and He responded. I will not attempt to talk you into or out of anything, but I will offer you H-O-P-E. I want my experience to encourage and empower you.

God's intent manifests in our lives when our intent agrees with His, which He expresses throughout His Word and quite concisely in 3 John 1:2: *Beloved, I pray that you may prosper in every way and [that your body] may keep well, even as [I know] your soul keeps well and prospers"*.

We will look at practical ways to pray with proper intent as well as practical ways to steward our recovered health. As we set forth, my prayer for you is the Apostle Paul's prayer in Ephesians 1:17-21:

> *God of our Lord Jesus, the Anointed, Father of Glory, I call out to You on behalf of Your people. Give them minds ready to receive wisdom and revelation so they will truly know You. Open the eyes of their hearts, and let the light of Your truth flood in. Shine Your light on the hope You are calling them to embrace. Reveal to them the glorious riches You are preparing as their inheritance. Let them see the full extent of Your power that is at work in those of us who believe, and may it be done according to Your might and power.*[1] (The Voice Translation)

Be encouraged! Throughout this book we focus on practical action to live in health and NEVER focus on doing something to avoid dying. Please stop for a moment and consider the difference between these two perspectives - the first is rooted in faith and the second in fear. Again, my goal is boldly slamming the door on cancer and locking such disease out of life rather than learning to live as long as possible with cancer (or any other disease).

Section I

Embracing the Healing Power of the Spirit

For though we walk (live) in the flesh, we are not carrying on our warfare according to the flesh and using mere human weapons.

For the weapons of our warfare are not physical [weapons of flesh and blood], but they are mighty before God for the overthrow and destruction of strongholds,

[Inasmuch as we] refute arguments and theories and reasonings and every proud and lofty thing that sets itself up against the [true] knowledge of God; and we lead every thought and purpose away captive into the obedience of Christ (the Messiah, the Anointed One),

2 Corinthians 10:3-5 (Amplified Version)

one

The Invitation

Welcome to the Emergency Room! I'm sure this is not the invitation you wanted to the place you most wanted to visit – especially as a patient. You know something is wrong but you don't know what it is. And a single visit may not get to the proper diagnosis. Maneuvering through the medical system of test after test, and prognosis after diagnosis is often a long and daunting journey. At first, those who are given a diagnosis of cancer feel like they've been given an invitation that leads to the gates of death. But it isn't true. The invitation is to choose life. And the outcomes can be beautiful. Cancer is not a final diagnosis. The power of life and death lie within you as you co-labor with the One who created you. Let me share how I learned this truth.

When I first walked into the Emergency Room, frustrated that routine tests had heretofore failed to give me answers, my anxiety made me hyper-alert to everyone around me. Did the Emergency Room receptionist look up and sigh when I walked through the door or did I project my own frustration onto her? I'm certain I had become a "thorn in the side" of the ER staff although my own exasperation at repeated inconclusive "work-ups" was beginning to surface. What was going on?

I would experience yo-yo blood pressure changes with an assortment of other alarming symptoms which absolutely convinced the medical staff that my problem was cardiac, yet I'd passed a myriad of cardiac tests. Once when hospitalized overnight for observation, my case had sparked a fairly heated bedside debate between a female attending physician and a male resident native to a country where women are little honored. He insisted, "It's all in her mind" in a demeaning tone. I was becoming "old news" and felt sure I was the last person anyone wanted to see walk in that ER door again. Yet, every time I did so, the measurable symptoms prompted considerable scurrying around and head scratching. This unproductive drill was wearing thin.

When the symptoms manifested one weekday morning while my husband was at work, my daughter insisted upon accompanying me to the ER. A gifted attorney, she understands objectively gathering and assessing information while maintaining a constructive persistence. Her skills helped me break the routine diagnostic cycle by tactfully insisting on changing the perspective regarding my case. We thought it logical to assume the cardiac route was played out and the search needed a whole body focus.

When the Emergency Room Chief again shrugged his shoulders about the non-results of another day-long effort, we politely questioned whether an earlier CT scan had included my abdomen which seemed reasonable considering I'd consistently reported being treated in that facility for a highly inflamed colon just two years previously. The condition had been due to over treatment with antibiotics from a misread routine colonoscopy. The chief admitted that the current scan had not included abdomen and agreed it was a logical pursuit. Finally, it was done, but I was admitted overnight awaiting results. My first meal in 12 hours was a well "aged" sandwich and a bottle of water. I was exhausted, frustrated, and dehydrated. Hospitals can be tough on a person's health.

The next morning the nurses were particularly cheerful - even chatty although evasive about the scan results saying, "The doctors have to give you those." I was not allowed to eat or drink until the doctors came by. Nurses grew apologetic as the day wore on with no doctor appearing.

Finally, mid-afternoon, a Chinese intern who I thought looked about fifteen years old shuffled into my room staring at the floor while he nervously revealed, "You have a mass in your pancreas." His words sucked all the air out of the room while a high voltage shiver went through my body. I sensed my husband trying to right his ship. "Where did this come from?" As numbness overtook panic, I was whisked off for even more scans, and my husband scurried out to consult with a surgeon friend and to call our grown children.

Somehow, on the way to the Radiology Department, it helped to focus on comforting this young sleep deprived intern since mine was obviously his first "C word" announcement. I made a weak joke that he had drawn the "short straw" for this assignment. He couldn't make eye contact. Once alone in the scan tube, I said a foxhole prayer, "Lord, I really don't know what else to say except to promise you that if you get me through this I will do my very best for You for the rest of my life." I meant it, and, amazingly, I realized He knew I did. It didn't feel like "let's make a deal". It was my first head on glimpse at the "main and the plain" of life even though it was not my first serious health battle. While I faced some excruciating challenges, I had no idea that the coming ordeal would lead me to some amazingly joyful and empowering revelations.

Later that evening an attending surgeon came by to say, "It looks like the "kind" of pancreatic cancer you have is a type that is usually slower growing." However, he said it could be locally aggressive and this one had already invaded surrounding tissue including a major vein to the colon (superior mesenteric vein) where that vein branches to the liver (portal vein). Then he casually assured that, even though surgery would necessitate removing my spleen, "You don't need it anyway." Of course they would also remove part of the pancreas, but his upbeat demeanor changed when he admitted the superior mesenteric vein was a serious concern. According to media reports, this is the same "kind of tumor" a famous computer executive, who obviously had every resource available to him, has since battled unsuccessfully. This "kind of tumor" isn't "statistically" considered to be highly metastatic as it more often spreads regionally.

Tumors apparently don't care much about medical statistics, and I would soon learn much about the dependability of pre and post surgery speculations. I was also beginning a very different journey than the predicted; "We'll cut it all out and just keep an eye on it". My foxhole prayer was certainly answered as the Lord met me where I was then wisely and lovingly led me, a latent Christian, out of "the valley of the shadow of death" miraculous step by miraculous step - often equipping me just in time to withstand an impending assault.

Tumor Location Does Not Explain WHAT Cancer Is.

I came to consider the absurdity of the term, "kind of cancer". When the tumor lives within you, "kind" is meaningless. The answer we need is to the question "what the heck IS cancer" regardless of location. In many decades of moving in medical circles, I had witnessed many discussions of cancer yet I recall zero discussion of **what it really is**. Being used to the world of specialized medicine, I suppose I simply accepted that various organ tissues might each manifest a "different kind" of cancer. Yet, I'd seen enough people struggle through chemotherapy and radiation to realize orthodox treatments impacted the entire person--body mind, and spirit. So many cancer patients I'd known "just wanted it **all** over with" rather than enduring yet more treatment. Within my cancer journey, I saw too many such cases in oncology waiting rooms like the frail, weary, pale woman wearing a scarf on her bald head who announced openly, "I wish I could opt for assisted suicide". Norman Cousins, who overcame terminal disease using unorthodox means, points out: "Drugs are not always necessary. Belief in recovery is." [1]

I will explain shortly how my own cancer journey eventually forced me to do an enormous amount of research regarding underlying origins of this insidious disease. There's more information available than one might imagine; therefore, I began to wonder why the public does not demand to be better informed. When someone tells you "you have cancer" and they want to cut, burn or poison the life out of it (along with the damaging the life force in the rest of your body), why shouldn't they explain what the origin of the disease is? Is compartmentalized medical science unable to embrace the whole organism?

Perhaps so, and I haven't yet taken you to the events in my own story where I realized there were important questions to ask that seemed to puzzle doctors. The story I've shared so far regards the first of two separate rounds of tumor surgery in my cancer saga. I have led you into the first round which I call "strike one". After this surgery, doctors reported we had "dodged a bullet". I had my life back. The trouble was, that particular life had allowed cancer to get a foothold in my body, and, although I did not understand at the time, "cutting it all" out could not change the part of that life that propagated cancer. Even if the oncologist and I had caved in to the surgeon's push for me to receive "off label" chemotherapy or, for that matter, if there had been a perfect chemotherapy available, it could not have cured the cause of this cancer. Cancer never just happens and, as I hope you see later in my story, understanding this fact is an essential first step toward slamming the door on this disease.

After my "strike one" surgery, my lifestyle changed little. Frankly, I didn't yet realize the impact of lifestyle on cancer. The doctors told me I could eat anything I wanted, and the oncologist, also a vintner, highly recommended red wine (rich in sugar), which I enjoyed. I had no idea that sugar is "cancer fertilizer", and, because most of my life I had carried a few extra pounds, I felt quite smug "keeping my weight up" per doctor's orders.

Even though surgery had been more complicated and recovery more challenging than expected, I believed I was back to normal within a year except for "keeping an eye on it" with tumor marker blood tests and CT Scans twice yearly.

Between twelve and eighteen months after "strike one" surgery, I experienced two traumatic events. First, I had a strange bout with a stubborn and severe tooth abscess "requiring" strong systemic IV antibiotics. Second, I was blindsided by a jolting conflict with a family member leaving me extremely offended and emotionally wounded. It was one of many such episodes occurring over decades that consistently evoked profound feelings of helplessness. I recall taking a long lonely walk after this particular encounter and desperately praying for strength and honestly caring little, at that point, whether I lived or died. Yet, it never entered my mind that either of these terribly stressful "insults" (please remember that word) might trigger a cancer relapse. After all, the surgeons had "gotten it all" and consistently clear follow-ups seemed to verify their assessment.

Foxhole Faith

Perhaps you've noticed, by now, that I was still far better at foxhole praying than more mature Scriptural prayer. Oh, I had sincerely thanked God for the success of my first surgery and I had picked up a Bible and started reading Psalms, but I didn't have a clue why I was compelled to do so. My religious past included being very actively raised in a church yet I had somehow escaped Scriptural understanding. Since college, I had very little energy for "religion" and certainly no concept of prayer beyond polite general monologues and panicked emergency requests. Over the years, I'd managed to slip in a few requests for wisdom and strength at particularly difficult times believing it improper to bother God with my puny life issues. I believe you will come to see why I'm very grateful that, within my cancer experience, I learned that God is not to blame for either disease or religion and He is concerned about every single thing that concerns you and me. The very moment I realized that He actually knows my name, my prayer life soared to say nothing of an explosion in my healing energy. As I weave my own story into this book, I believe you will see God's heart and hand in that story. He put people in my life who taught me powerful ways to pray which I will later share.

I'm compelled to disclose that learning to pray Scripturally has been empowering in many ways including interceding for others - even those unaware of that intercession. I have prayerfully interceded for the family member I spoke of earlier. Their own wounded soul, often manifesting in anger management issues, has been healed so that the difficult conflicts have subsided. Oh that I would have known, before cancer, that "religion" does not equal relationship with a God who wants to dialogue with us! Please understand that intercession must be done Scripturally. I am not talking about manipulating people to suit our own agendas. I'm talking about compassionately applying the blood and resurrection power of Jesus to a wounded soul. We will expand this discussion later, and, I pray, you will see how prayer tunes us into God so that He can disclose to us what we must do to lock cancer, indeed to lock disease, out of our lives.

Let's settle something before we move on. I am keenly aware that many believers and non-believers are confused about whether or not God wants every single person healed in body, soul and spirit which follows that they doubt He wants us all "in health". We need to put this doubt aside now because it is a very real block to the manifestation of our healing. We will later discuss how our healing is a "done deal" through the finished work of Jesus. For now, please keep two things in mind. Scripture tells us that Jesus healed every single person **who came to Him** for healing. It also teaches us *"Jesus is the same yesterday, today, and forever"*. (Hebrews 13:8) In her book, *Heal Them All,* Rev. Cheryl Schang writes: **"Jesus healed them all!** We are at a crossroads here. **Jesus healed them all!** Every time, always, everyone, whosoever, whatsoever, totally, wholly, completely, thoroughly - He healed them all. Now if it is not God's will for all of them to be healed, was Jesus in rebellion? Jesus was not in rebellion because it is God's will to heal every single time - ALL." [2]

I'm aware there are a number of passages in Scripture often taught to make excuses for circumstances in which it might appear that God did not choose to heal someone. I will not delve into a theological discussion about these. Rev. Schang's book (among others listed in Appendix Two) does an exquisite job explaining these passages and I HIGHLY recommend reading it. For now, I ask you to consider that, "People who think that God does not want to heal may have limited the concept of healing to an instant miracle. Recovery is a process, not an event." [3] My own story, which I describe as an "interactive miracle" was quite a process; therefore, please put aside your doubt about God's will to see you "in health" at this point so that it does not distract you from starting your own process of healing. Doubt was my own worst enemy, as you will soon learn.

Don't Panic!

It took an unfortunate relapse I share later for me to realize what counselor, Gary Sinclair, cleverly expresses in his book, *Your Empowering Spirit*, saying, "We live in La Lar Land waiting for someone else to sprinkle Foo Fue dust upon us to make everything all right without realizing that the answers do not lie without, they lie within." [4] I started out believing my healing would come from the familiar medical culture; however, my journey forced me to learn a great deal that is apparently not taught in medical school. I came to realize that, if we know the underlying cause(s) of cancer, then we can get past what I consider the compromising goal of "remission" and move toward slamming the door on cancer, locking it out, and completing a beautiful life.

I also learned that the answer absolutely is within and is activated when we allow God's ever present Spirit to move within our very being. Holy Spirit is a gentleman yearning and waiting for an invitation to colabor with us. We have free will to say "yes" or "no" to God, but "sort of" and "sometimes" are not options. When we ask, He never says "No". There are a lot of contrived "new" spiritual paradigms that fear driven seekers are grasping for because they worry they will have to give up part of their lives if they submit to God. Guess what! The "things" we need to give up are the things that make us sick and we are freed from them when we truly trust God. God set up ALL the systems of natural or universal law to work for our joy. He makes it very clear that we can choose to operate within these systems or not as Deuteronomy 30:19 discloses:

> *I call heaven and earth to witness this day against you that I have set before you life and death, the blessings and the curses; therefore choose life, that you and your descendants may live.*

Apparently for a lot of people, including nominal Christians, knowing the location of a tumor is enough information on which to base life or death choices even without getting additional information or opinions - especially God's opinion. Driven by fear and panic we just want that thing out of there a.s.a.p! "Somebody bring the pink Foo Fue dust and hurry!" I knew this undermining fear and panic all too well from the moment I first heard the "C Word" pertaining to my own body. Somehow, through the initial fear, God heard my honest, simple foxhole prayer spoken **before** I made treatment decisions and my miracle began at that very point. I had a deep hole to climb out of and had no intention of hanging around the edge once I reached daylight. I wasn't about to settle for "remission" or treatments that I'd watched suck the life force out of so many others. I had long thought of most cancer treatments as sort of like whacking your foot with a sledgehammer to get rid of an ingrown toenail. These treatments just did not make sense to me and even fear and panic didn't change that fact.

I have never understood "remission" as a goal because the very word imparts fear of relapse, which, to me, seems like settling for temporary health. Choosing life, I believe, means that I choose total healing. I realized that the power of my thoughts and words would cause me to either settle into partial life/partial death (remission), or total health and the fullness of life. So, I set aside the medical terminology and focused on God's presence and His Word. Throughout my battle, I was very careful to never speak or allow others to speak the word, "remission".

Choosing life means not just seeking healing for cancer. Life involves your body, mind and spirit.

Who You Know Trumps What You Know

I am well aware that cancer can send you crawling through the minefield of your own imagination. You can have many well-meaning people surrounding you but you are alone because they "have lives" and yours is "on hold" at best. Many times early in my cancer battle, the enemy of my soul kept me busy dodging his "flaming darts" or negative accusing thoughts. At that time I had only a dusty little "shield of faith" (see Ephesians 6:16) to fend them off. A ruthless accuser and liar, satan brings stuff like, "Why would you be healed when so many other better people than you have died of cancer?" "God is mad at you. You know you've given

Him good reason." At that particular time I knew so little Scripture that it seemed like this enemy made good points. I had no clue how to *"take every thought captive"* or even that I needed to do so (2 Corinthians 10:5).

Early one morning after days of such attacks, my eyes literally popped open from a sound sleep, and, immediately, I heard quite audibly (at least to me), "The Bible is true." And, the strange thing is, I knew that I knew that I knew, right then and there, that it is true. I didn't even think the experience was odd. Immediately I was holding the biggest sword in the universe--God's Word. My dusty little shield of faith was suddenly gleaming. I still didn't know much Scripture, but I was highly motivated to change that fact because, if you have virtual truth, what can hurt you? I was about to become a close personal friend of Him who is the *"Word made flesh"* (John 1:14) and who is *"The Way, the TRUTH, and the Life"* (John 14:6). Who you know is always more important than what you know. I would never be alone again. Panic left me.

Once panic withdrew, I became determined to know how I could beat this diagnosis. If only I could learn about the roots of cancer, I could surely slam the door on it through my knowledge and the resulting steps I would take to change my body-mind and make it healthy and whole. It dawned on me through this totally unanticipated revelation I just shared that what I would come to know depended totally upon my interaction with the Master Physician, the One who created each of us and can recreate us, Our Healer.

The Enemy is NOT God!

Even if you know little Scripture, you have probably heard the story of David, the shepherd boy, and Goliath, the giant champion of an evil pagan nation; a story told in 1 Samuel 17. The Israelites are cowering in their battle camp for weeks and David shows up with supplies for his older brothers. He is appalled when Goliath comes out repeatedly taunting the Israelite army by demanding they choose a champion of their own to fight him "winner take all". Asking, *"who is this uncircumcised Philistine that he should defy the army of the living God?"* (1 Samuel 17:26). David, who has protected a sheep herd against ferocious wild animals using only a sling and stones shuns the king's offer of his own armor, gathers five smooth river stones, and runs TOWARD the mocking giant using his sling to sink a stone in the giant's forehead. Then he took Goliath's own sword and severed the giant's head. (This part of the story is really important because if we cut the head off the bully, cancer, the rest of the disease must follow.) Then, seeing that David had be-headed their champion, all the Philistines turned and withdrew because they had met their match in a mere boy, but a boy who had an intimate relationship with the Creator of the Universe developed through a lot of dialogue with God while out in the fields.

I share this story because we need to keep our enemy and our God in perspective. Before we delve into how science and Scripture converge and consider the practical aspects of fighting cancer, we need to consider specifically what cancer IS NOT and, conversely, what cancer IS. We need to know the enemy that taunts us in order to make us fearful even though *"God did not give us a spirit of fear, but of power, and of love, and of a sound mind."* (2 Timothy 1:7, YLT) We also need at least a cursory overview of our internal environment where this insidious enemy sets up camp to bully us. And we need to remember that we can beat this enemy because we, like David, are aligned with the living God and He provides **all** that we need when we faithfully co-labor with Him.

Cancer Myths:

Cancer is the subject of many frightening myths. And it cannot be dissected away from your body in an instant. Because the body is connected to our minds and to our thoughts and our spirit, we must take a whole person approach to healing. As we begin discussing "whole body health", don't be intimidated but rather be encouraged by the complexity of what Psalm 139:14 refers to as the *"fearfully and wonderfully made"* human body and soul (mind, will, emotions). The prophet, Hosea, who reported God's observation: *"My people perish for lack of knowledge"* (Hosea 4:6) helps us to understand that only the Creator has ALL that knowledge we need for healing. However, we can understand the "pure laws of health" that merge science with God's Word. In that understanding, we gain powerful insight into disease - specifically cancer. And especially, what cancer is not.

Cancer is not:

- ❖ the result of unchangeable DNA.
- ❖ something that just happens.
- ❖ punishment from God.
- ❖ a compulsory death sentence.
- ❖ incurable.

Cancer IS NOT the result of unchangeable DNA.

Did you know that you can change your DNA to slam the door on cancer? Dr. Bruce Lipton, PhD, in his book, *The Biology of Belief*, describes epigenetics as "the new science of self-empowerment. . . The term, 'epigenetics' literally means 'control above genetics'." [5] "It is the science of how environmental signals select, modify, and regulate gene activity. This new awareness reveals that our genes are constantly being remodeled in response to life experiences. Which again emphasizes that our perceptions of life shape our biology." [6] As we move through learning how to tune into God so He can tell us what to do in our lives to lock out cancer, I believe we can be encouraged by knowing that He absolutely created us to heal when we fully cooperate with His plans for us. Our bodies have amazing healing power as my own story illustrates.

Dr. Lipton also reports, "In the last decade, epigenetic research has established that DNA blueprints passed down through genes are not set in concrete at birth. Genes are not destiny! Environmental influences, including nutrition, stress, and emotions, can modify those genes without changing their basic blueprint. And those modifications, epigeneticists have discovered, can be passed on to future generations as surely as DNA blueprints are passed on via the double helix." [7]

If you want to dig deeper into the insights of epigenetics regarding cancer, Lipton works through some studies and cites others. I was encouraged to read, "The malignancies in a significant number of cancer patients are derived from environmentally induced epigenetic alterations and not defective genes." [8]

Biblically speaking, the "natural science" of epigenetics would seem invaluable in illustrating the dynamics of "generational curses" and add to our realization that healing of the body can be blocked until we are healed of specific wounds upon our souls or past traumas as well as being released from specific soul ties with other human beings like old lovers. We will later look at specific strategies for healing our souls to remove very real blocks to healing of our bodies.

Cancer IS NOT "Something That Just Happens" or "Bad Luck"

The belief that "cancer is something that just happens" or, worse, that "cancer is punishment from God" may be the product of ignorance, frustration, or erroneous religious doctrine. In some ways, these concepts seek to excuse "perishing for lack of knowledge" or not "standing up and fighting". Almost always, they are the rationalization for confusing circumstances around us rather than the realization of God's truth or the understanding of even the most basic science regarding lifestyle and attitudes including the impact of our own thoughts and words upon our health. By the time you finish this book, I intend for you to better understand the insidious nature of cancer, which I consider to be the "Goliath" of disease.

Sometimes, the emotional need to rationalize "getting cancer" leads to various forms of "victim mentality". In this process, we can unknowingly embrace the "drama of the trauma" which may dangerously feed negative energy into our mind, will and emotion (our soul). We will view in depth the important topic of verbally declaring our healing later, but I need to make the point early on that we must be very careful who we discuss our diagnosis with and even who we ask to pray for us. We do NOT need sympathy! We need compassion, which Jesus modeled perfectly by doing something to change the situation. The enemy may try to use our own loved ones against us in insidious ways if they are caught up in fear or don't understand God's perfect will for healing.

Another precaution I took was to avoid looking up statistics online even when doctors suggested doing so. Statistics mean NOTHING! I won't waste ink on the thousands of reasons why except to say that statistics are tools for furthering agendas, period. A lot of online "sites" are remission minded sympathy sites so I carefully avoided those. I started my blog, www.realhealthhope.com as an alternative to such sites. There are many well-meaning movements in place to "promote cancer awareness". As we later consider how our focus influences reality, we may want to re-think participation in such movements. I am uncomfortable with cancer awareness as an impetus for celebration. Cancer is of the enemy and he loves attention any way he can get it and cancer as a brand is, in my mind, counterproductive. I suggest "health awareness".

Some cancer treatment centers try to set up connections between current patients and "survivors" although volunteers may be required to walk on spiritual eggshells and temper their encouragement to avoid "false hope" - whatever that is. Remember the enemy of our souls is not creative, but he is a master at counterfeit support even in the most well meaning among us. We will discuss further the important difference between sympathy and compassion as well as how to pray effectively for healing to manifest. For now, I again stress that it is critical to realize that God wants us not merely "in remission" but "in health". Now might be a good time to stop and read Psalms 103. By the way "every" means "every" and "all" means "all". I never describe myself as a "cancer survivor". I am healed of pancreatic cancer, period.

Cancer is NOT Punishment from God

Jesus participated in countless healing miracles. He never pre-judged whether a person was or was not "worthy" of healing. Again, He healed every single person who came to Him seeking healing. Jesus sometimes told the healed person "not to tell anyone". Occasionally, Jesus would not even let all the disciples be around Him when he healed or delivered someone. As I've learned more about quantum physics, I have wondered if at least one reason He told the healed not to tell anyone was that He realized their faith was not yet full and He did not want the negative energy vibrations of other people's doubt in the atmosphere. Or perhaps He didn't want observers judging the sick person's worthiness because, in the culture of that day, sickness was commonly considered punishment for personal sin.

Jesus sometimes took a person aside to heal them as in Mark 8:23 and 7:31, or He sent the doubters and mourners away from a healing scene as in the case of Jairus' daughter where they actually laughed at Him in Luke 8:51-53:

> *And when He came to the house, He permitted no one to enter with Him except Peter and John and James, and the girl's father and mother.*
> *And all were weeping for and bewailing her; but He said, Do not weep, for she is not dead but sleeping.*
> *And they laughed Him to scorn, knowing full well that she was dead.*

Doubt is an enemy ploy to distract us and weaken our resolve. I cannot overemphasize the importance of surrounding yourself with positive energy. I don't know exactly how it all works, but Scripturally, scientifically and in my own experience, the positive energy of "believing believers" who actually believe God rather than merely believing IN God is absolutely integral to having one's healing manifest whether immediately or over time.

There was a time, in my "strike two" recovery, which was far more difficult than the "strike one" recovery, when God used a very practical interchange with my family to illustrate my point. I asked my family to upgrade my basic walker to one with a seat because I often became exhausted just dragging from my chair to the bathroom. They put off my request, and instead, they agreed in a kindly matter-of-fact way, "You aren't going to be on that walker very long anyway. You are getting stronger every time you stand up." It may have seemed a bit insensitive at the time, but I needed to hear that they believed in my healing progress. Of course, God was at work in their tough love. My family was correct because I was soon moving about without any walker.

At another moment when I was beginning to weaken in my resolve, God Himself admonished me with words audible to my soul saying, "Stand Up and Fight!" This came at a point when I was tired of feeling helpless and exhausted - okay it was a pity party. At that Rhema (spoken) word from God, I knew I was not alone and I had an assigned part to play in my healing. I hit my knees and, in the attitude of Queen Esther, prayed in Esther 4:16: "Lord, If I perish, I perish, but I am giving it ALL to You. I will stand leaning against YOU! I trust YOU! I love YOU! I know You love me and that is a new thing for me because a few months ago I didn't even realize you knew my name." Very clearly, in my spirit, I heard the words spoken to Joshua and others repeatedly in the Old Testament, *"Be strong and courageous"* and *"I will be with you."* (See Joshua 1.) Joshua had a lot of fighting to do, but, like David, he NEVER did it under his own power. This message is practical truth and I hope you meditate on it. I've never had to fight the cancer bully alone nor will you. You could never have done anything to "deserve" a dose of cancer as punishment from a God who IS love. You could never DO anything to deserve that love and the healing power in it, but it is yours. The enemy is the source of sickness and God is health. As the Apostle James writes: *Submit yourselves therefore to God. Resist the devil, and he **will** flee from you.* (James 4:7, KJV)

As Cal Pierce, director of Healing Rooms International, says in his strong teaching, "Destroying Cancer": "The enemy has no power or authority. Fear gives him a license to use our power." [9] Some people are afraid to boldly seek the manifestation of their healing because they have been taught wrong interpretations of Old Testament Covenant passages and believe, like Jesus's contemporaries did, that God will curse you with sickness for breaking covenant and doing any of the things on the "law list" in Deuteronomy 28. If you need to correct this teaching, I again highly recommend Rev. Cheryl Schang's book, *Heal Them All* and Marilyn Hickey's book, *Be Healed*. But let me share an important kernel of God's truth. Blessings and curses, part of the Old Covenant, are misunderstood both when taken out of historical context and when discernment of the New Covenant is lacking. As Galatians 3:13 succinctly teaches, Jesus hung on the tree to *"become a curse for us"* so we are NOT cursed with cancer by our sin. If we accept the finished work of Christ, we are NOT subject to that curse of sin-consciousness and sickness. (NO! This is not a license to sin; drink this truth in and you won't be compelled to sin or you will be honestly and cathartically repentant if you happen to.) Old Testament Scripture is not generally accurate literal basis for forming healing doctrine. We have a New Testament; a New Covenant. It is a legal document and it starts with the finished work of Christ and we are the heirs.

Cancer IS NOT "incurable"

Cancer is also not "incurable" although the idea that the cure must come from either a complex scientific discovery, silver bullet supplement, or pink "Foo Foo Dust" is not well founded. The enemy of our souls would like us to believe that, once cancer is diagnosed, the end is pretty much a matter of time unless some sort of instantaneous miracle occurs or medical science has that big breakthrough. Henry W. Wright states, "When you say 'incurable', you have made the devil greater than God." [10] Our already defeated bully certainly needs us to believe this lie if he has any chance of taking us out. He wants us to believe we are helpless and alone both scientifically and spiritually. It is a lie! As reported in John 10:10: *The thief comes only in order to steal and kill and destroy. I (Jesus) came that they may have and enjoy life, and have it in abundance (to the full, till it overflows).*

We must always size up our enemy through the lens of THE truth—Jesus Christ.

It is pertinent that in the John 10:10 Scripture, "steal" is listed before "kill" and "destroy". Why would Holy Spirit, who does nothing by accident, put steal before kill? What is the enemy trying to steal? He wants to remove the Word of God from within our hearts! He knows the power of that Word even more than many believers do--when we speak God's own Word, grace and power come with it. If satan can steal the Word, he can kill. It's that simple. All Scripture is *"God breathed"* (2 Timothy 3:16). Holy Spirit is saying our defeated enemy would like to steal the only offensive weapon the Apostle Paul listed in the "full armor of God":

Finally, be strong in the Lord and in his mighty power.
Put on the full armor of God so that you can take your stand against the devil's schemes.
For our struggle is not against flesh and blood, but against the rulers, against the authorities, against the powers of this dark world and against the spiritual forces of evil in the heavenly realms.
Therefore put on the full armor of God, so that when the day of evil comes, you may be able to stand your ground, and after you have done everything, to stand.
Stand firm then, with the belt of truth buckled around your waist, with the breastplate of righteousness in place,
and with your feet fitted with the readiness that comes from the gospel of peace.
In addition to all this, take up the shield of faith, with which you can extinguish all the flaming arrows of the evil one.
Take the helmet of salvation and the sword of the Spirit, which is the word of God.
(Ephesians 6:10-17, NIV, my)

Again, the enemy of our souls wants to steal the truth, the Word of God, from us so we replace our faith with fear and then hang around waiting for someone else to run at our giant for us. Satan is the enemy of our souls because his only weapon is the planting of negative thoughts in our soul. I've mentioned the power of words and thoughts several times. In future chapters, we will look more closely at how to deal with the assault on our souls as a critical part of our healing process. It is this insidious assault that often explains why we lose so many to cancer who appear to be living "beautiful lives".

Just as dark cannot remain within light, fear cannot remain within faith. Our words activate **either** fear or faith - never both.

I find it fascinating and pertinent that not only is the Word of God the only offensive weapon "issued" with the "armor of God" in the Ephesians 6, but ALL the "body armor" in this Scripture covers the front of the warrior. God's armor is designed to protect those who **stand and fight** or, like David, run **toward** the attacking enemy of their souls. As Henry W. Wright says, "Our backsides are vulnerable if we turn and run". [11] I have found both the truth and imagery of this Scripture quite empowering. Later, when we look at quantum science, I will share an amazing experience I had by standing and wielding the "sword of the Spirit" when I was under very real and very serious symptomatic attack just two weeks before I was scheduled for a follow up CT scan after my surgery. I will continue to share how I "cancer-ed myself" and how God led me to "uncancer myself". Let's take a closer look at the mechanisms that can "cancer" us.

Cancer Truths:

Once we understand what cancer is not, we begin to face the facts of cancer more realistically – without fear. And when you see what cancer is attached to, you can begin to change the environment of your body to fight. Basically, I came to see that cancer is a response of our body cells and includes:

- ❖ body cells responding to an imbalanced "inner terrain"
- ❖ the ultimate cellular level response to overwhelming toxin intake
- ❖ the ultimate cellular level response to undersupply of essential building and maintenance materials

Cancer is body cells responding to an imbalanced "inner environment"

Compare body cells to fish in an aquarium totally dependent upon us to keep their environment clean and balanced. Our "inner environment" has chemical and electrical aspects. A great benefit of our *"fearfully and wonderfully made bodies"* (Psalm 139:14) is that we do not need to fully understand our inner complexities to "be in health" just as I don't have to be a "computer geek" to get the most benefit from my laptop computer. Rather, my efficient enjoyment of it directly correlates to my not defiling it with corrupt input and careless maintenance. I honor its complexities with good care and it serves me according to its design.

As Henry W. Wright says, **"A healthy cell will never become cancerous."** [12] When I was forced to "become my own doctor," Wright's statement also occurred to me. It just made sense that, if I could return my body cells to full blown health, cancer would have no place to set up camp in my body. A bully only attacks the weak. So, I set about to discover what made a body cell weak or unhealthy so I could reverse the process. In future chapters we look even more specifically at what I learned; however, the underlying precept depends upon balancing the "inner terrain" physically, mentally, and emotionally.

Cancer is the ultimate cellular level response to overwhelming toxin intake

What is a toxin? It's poison and it can be thoughts, words, foods, or environmental elements! Chemotherapy is actually an example of toxins purposely administered to kill cells. Social media and the Internet are filled with information about environmental toxins. We do need to actively avoid environmental toxins; however, sometimes "toxin hype" does little more than spread fear to push an ideological agenda. I consciously avoid toxic fear because worry, itself, is a sin - essentially an emotional toxin because it is an effort to nullify something within our innate design. Sin is purposefully doing what will defile body, mind, and spirit--but we can also defile ourselves out of ignorance. Many good people are ignorant of fear as a defiling sin. Science has shown that sustained fear actually has a negative effect on the immune system. In Scripture, the much-referenced Job, who dealt with tremendous personal calamity, (that some try to blame on God) admitted that his own fear attracted *"that which he had feared most"* (Job 3:35). Job was describing the natural "Law of Attraction". Quantum mechanics teaches the same lesson explaining that energy flows where we pay attention and what we intend creates the end result.

We must be aware of toxins to avoid in our environment - but to do so constructively. A simple rule is: Choose what you use in the form closest to that which God made it, and, whenever possible, avoid highly "processed", contrived, or "refined" substances starting with food and drink but including soap, cosmetics and cleaning materials. It actually applies to every material and substance we use.

Of course we will visit this subject again in detail. For now, please realize that we can greatly improve our health by managing toxin intake including that from our environment, our interaction with others, and our lifestyle choices. Again, we are created with defense systems in place to deal with a certain level of toxins; however, there is a toxin limit that we must respect in order to maintain a steady "healthy state". We should reserve that toxin limit for emergencies and avoid knowingly using it for destructive eating, drinking, thinking, etc. If we are already in a "disease state", of course it is critical to detoxify without adding to the already stressed defense systems in our bodies. As Hippocrates is often quoted as saying about medical treatment, "first do no harm".

Cancer is the ultimate cellular level response to under-supply of essential building and maintenance materials

"Living healthy" is often viewed as denying ourselves of things we enjoy: food, drink, and entertainment. Such a perspective of denial is toxic in itself because "will power" and holding to a list of rigid don'ts is operating from weakness (a worldly view) rather than strength (a perspective of where we stand from God's Kingdom view). A healthier focus targets what we "get to do" that makes us feel incredibly and sustainably energetic, mentally alert, emotionally peaceful, physically vigorous, joyful, and optimistic. I might also add that self-control becomes second nature when we move **toward** a visualized beneficial goal rather than struggling to move **away** from something we are tied to in an unhealthy way.

In other words, when our bodies get a fresh steady supply of good groceries, water, emotional stimuli, oxygen, joy, and rest, we feel so incredibly good we are increasingly drawn to those habits and the choices that enhance that feeling. Our cells need what "we" need and its been discovered that, on our cell membranes, there are receptors for "molecules of emotion" customized to receive specific molecules such as insulin, endorphins, etc. Interestingly, the natural life pro-moting endorphins (feel good molecules) fit the same receptors as life destroying opiate drugs. When healthy, we create our own natural and productive "feel good drugs". I have felt better in my post cancer lifestyle than ever before.

Give a body cell only what it needs day in and day out and it will be healthy. If it is healthy, the entire body-mind is healthy. Nothing "pre-vents" or "cures" disease like health. I urge you to meditate on that state-ment for a while. This realization was germane to my "un-cancering myself", as Cyberphysiologist Gary Sinclair terms the healing process, and remains so in enjoying a healthy state of being.

As I researched for survival, I realized that we cannot separate our cells from our "selves". And we cannot separate our "selves" from our Creator and enjoy wholeness. Tuning into God for our specific health plan is a must. As we receive the love of God and **listen** for His plan to restore our health, we realize that there is an enemy who sows seeds of destruction, but interactive faith in God sows seeds of love, joy, peace, patience, kindness, goodness, faithfulness, gentleness and **self-control** (Galatians 5:22-23). God created each of us in His image, and will restore us. It begins with opening up to His love and compassionate care which is very much like increasing the bandwidth of our souls so we can receive God's downloads meant just for us individually.

Notes:

two

The Spiritual Side to Healing

The invitation to step into a beautiful life here on earth involves learning to partner with the God who created us, and then shifting into a spiritual perspective on health and wholeness. True healing and recovery of health involves pursuing life and being patient with the process. Along the journey towards health every area of life transforms. God becomes someone rather than something so that the spiritual side to healing becomes a steadying life force.

Between my first hearing "the C word" from the young intern and then awakening one morning to hear in my spirit, "the Bible is true", significant time passed. The tumor the intern announced was surgically removed along with the first one-third of my pancreas and my spleen. As I mentioned earlier, the tumor's invasion into a major vein was, indeed, a serious issue requiring a surprise second surgery a day before anticipated discharge. Recovery was complicated by this "double whammy".

Finally, I was told, "We got it all; eat whatever you want; keep your weight up and get on with life." I took that advice to heart not realizing that going on with the same life left the door wide open to a cancer relapse.

Surprise! And Sorry About Your Luck

The oncologist who followed up after what I call my "strike one surgeries (2)" was casual about following me until three scans later when a very large tumor popped up within just six months—a very large tumor that had already invaded the remaining pancreas, stomach, small colon, pyloric valve, and, yet again, the superior mesenteric vein. Later, a nuclear scan showed that the gall bladder was also "hot", and there were "spots" on my liver and lungs. A "non-aggressive slow growing kind of cancer?" Hardly!

The day the scans revealed this surprise tumor, the diagnosing doctors basically said, "sorry about your luck, it's absolutely inoperable".

Unlikely Seed of Hope is Planted Just in Time

Blindsided by this report, I drove home with my head spinning. But, amazingly, I had one seed of hope from something that miraculously happened into my life just days before this shock. The entire two weeks prior to this occurrence had actually set me up for a series of events I now realize began my "inter-active miracle". I couldn't recognize the synchronicity at first because miracles had never been part of my theology. Again, although I'd been active in church through college, my view of it was more like a community service organization. I thought that being a "good person", doing some "good works", and not breaking the Ten Commandments (at least the bad ones) was "the Christian life".

At church youth camp, I had been taught that I was third, behind God and others, and somehow warped that concept into being "a nice Christian girl". In the 1950's "nice girls" accepted their subordinate status. I believed that, even if it meant becoming a verbal punching bag for others, it was not appropriate to bother God praying about mundane events in my life. After all, who was I to ask for favor? Coincidentally, I've heard several other cancer patients say, "Who was I to pray for healing?" That kind of thinking is from the enemy at work because it certainly is NOT from God.

As I mentioned earlier, after my "strike one" tumor experience including my foxhole prayer, I had made no significant lifestyle changes except trying to pray my gratitude and rather generically asking for wisdom and strength. I was sincere, but I had no idea how to pray Scripturally standing on God's promises. Regarding diet and exercise, I didn't see a need to adjust anything at that time because the medical culture I'd married into decades earlier saw food as pretty much inert.

Still, that foxhole prayer in the CT scan tube after first hearing the "C word" certainly had been heard. God was already working on my behalf. Two days after undergoing the CT scan that would reveal the shocking relapse and three days before I received the scan results that forced me back into the "batter's box", a most unlikely human "angel" crossed my path. We were doing some back yard construction and needed a fence. I had seen one at a friend's home and was strangely compelled to have her contractor do our fence. The friend could only remember the man's last name. Uncharacteristically, I was so driven to find that contractor that I began to call everyone in the phone book with his last name asking if they had a fencing business. I found him and scheduled an estimate. Again uncharacteristically, I did not consider getting other estimates. I was getting on with life since scans had been "all clear" for 18 months.

The day the fencing contractor visited, a strange conversation occurred - at least for a business appointment. He measured the site and we sat down to look at fence style photos. When he opened his portfolio, a few snapshots fell out. He apologized because they were pictures of a bad car accident he had not meant to leave in the folder, but he said, "These are pictures of an accident that nearly killed my wife. Coincidentally, she has the same first name as you". He seemed strangely compelled to tell me the story and I found myself curiously mesmerized as he did.

His wife's car accident had landed her in the same university medical center where my "strike one" occurred. Only one day before he and the family were faced with discontinuing life support, his brother had called him from out of state to say, "I have a Scripture for you." Over the phone, he read from the book of James, chapter 5:14-15:

Is anyone among you sick? He should call in the church elders (the spiritual guides). And they should pray over him, anointing him with oil in the Lord's name. And the prayer [that is] of faith will save him, who is sick, and the Lord will restore him; and if he has committed sins, he will be forgiven.

The contractor, a recovering dormant Christian much like I was, had answered, "I don't know a minister much less any 'elders' who would do this for me." But his brother did know of a pastor who would help them and gave him the contact information.

Comfort Zone Adjustments Occur In Prayer

About this time I found myself thinking, "Oh boy, this is getting out of my comfort zone." Anointing with oil was a totally foreign concept to me. I was also struggling with the idea of depending on prayer of "elders" whoever they were. Even more indicative of my faith deficit was the fact that I did not even know there was a book of James in the Bible prior to the contractor sharing his story even though I'd been in church every time the door opened until a few years after college when a husband in medical residency and two children born within a span of 16 months had made slacking off easy.

Regardless of my comfort zone, the contractor seemed driven to continue saying, "I called the pastor who agreed to come pray for my wife. Coincidentally, when he came, another pastor of a church we had visited a few times showed up at the same time and they went to my wife's bedside, laid hands on her, prayed over her, and anointed her forehead with oil. I had told my children we were going to do this, but had cautioned them not to get their hopes up because of what the doctors said." He continued, "I have to admit I'd never been much on church and this was all new to me." Miraculously, the very next day his wife was sitting up in a chair feeding herself with no life support. Soon she was discharged from the hospital and, at this writing, is completely recovered not only from the accident but also from chronic spine issues she had suffered with previously.

I remember thinking, "what a nice story, but could we get back to the fence". At that point, I had no idea how important the contractor's story would become to me.

The very evening after receiving the news of my ominous "inoperable tumor", I called this fencing contractor who immediately had that same minister give me a call and we prayed right there on the phone which, before that day, would have seemed weird to me. Today, I still recall much of that prayer because it was so new to me to think that I could ask straight up for my healing to manifest even though I hadn't been living a particularly **religious** life for decades.

What Kind of Prayer is That?

I was soon to learn that God is not to blame for **religion**. One of the most memorable parts of the telephone prayer was the pastor reminding God by mentioning specific Scriptures of God's promises for healing in His Word. I recall thinking, "Wow, that's kind of bold." But there was power in the words and he had a tone of confidence.

Then, he prayed, "Lord, In the name of Jesus, I bind the enemy of her soul from further harming your daughter."

"Whoa!" I thought, "That's even bolder. Can he really do that?" Immediately, I felt lighter from sensing both weight lift off and darkness disperse. My healing journey had begun.

When Pastor Tom had finished his prayer, he invited me to the mid-week service at his church the following evening. He explained that he would call for those needing personal prayer to come to the altar after the service and he would basically follow James 5:13-14 then. The next twenty-four hours passed slowly and anxiously, but my fence contractor "angel" unexpectedly showed up in the midst of it ostensibly to check a couple of fence measurements. He took the opportunity to seed my faith by telling me of a number of other healing miracles within his family since his wife's recovery. I urge you to never underestimate the immense and essential power of testimony in building faith.

Wednesday night finally came and my husband and I went to church for the first time in quite a while. We had never heard a band play in church and certainly had never seen an altar call short of our own going forth as children to confess our faith prior to baptism. Pastor Tom came to our seats and warmly welcomed us before the service putting us both at ease.

When I walked to the alter after that service, the church elders placed their hands on me and the pastor put consecrated oil on my forehead while praying, again, according to Scripture. I recall that Pastor Tom actually commanded the tumor to die and my body to return to health. I literally heard clearly in my spirit, "An old life has ended and a new one has begun". This revelation was especially good news in light of something I had "heard" in my spirit during the difficult relationship conflict I mentioned earlier - an ominous, "Be still, this life is about to end". What I have learned about "soul wounds" since that time, which I will be sharing throughout this book, has clarified a great deal of this revelation.

I want to stop and share two important considerations about this important James 5 Scripture. Rev. Cheryl Schang explains that God wants us healed so much that, if we don't have our own faith, He will let us use someone else's faith. [1] Those who hold office of "church elder" are, by Biblical definition, supposed to be mature and sure in their Biblical faith. Schang is clear that those ministering (in this case elders) "are to be the ones with the faith, not necessarily the sick person. . . It is hard to have faith when you are sick and hurting." [2] I believe my own story illustrates this point. Now, what's the deal with the oil?

In Exodus 30, there are specific instructions for God's anointing oil that distinguishes it from oils pagans used in idolatry. Churches don't necessarily mix oil by that specific recipe now. In fact, the ingredients aren't readily available. However, churches pray to consecrate anointing oil which, when done with reverent intent, is quite capable of changing that oil in supernatural ways. Quantum Physics teaches us this dynamic and we know that words and intent change matter. The purpose of anointing with oil is still as God originally intended - it is the "contact point" between the anointed person and God, Himself, a point that cannot be duplicated. "God was/is saying, 'I have my own oil, and, when you mark somebody with that oil, you are marking them with the mark of Jehovah God, and I am obligated to them because they wear My mark; and they will be healed'." [3] The oil service is an act of obedience even though many

Christian churches overlook this Scripture and substitute a prayer list ritual. My own oil service experience was profound and has given me a "point of contact" to return to many times throughout my journey. I remember it vividly in my spirit.

A Vision is Worth a 1,000 Words

That night after the oil service, I fell asleep peacefully yet later abruptly awakened to a full color vision of my entire pancreas with profuse vividly colored fluids sizzling away from around it. I could even hear the sizzling. Signs and wonders had never been in my "faith package", but I was not alarmed at all by this experience. I realized that the bright yellow fluids in the vision were more the focus of the vision than the soft purple pancreas itself. There was no reasoning or puzzling about what I'd seen. I just fell back into peaceful sleep.

The next morning, I awakened knowing something within me had changed profoundly. I knew a miracle had occurred even though my tumor was still palpable from the surface. I soon realized I was without a familiar spirit of offense, which included bitterness, resentment, and anger that I had harbored since experiencing a terrible and avoidable health care trauma in my twenties.

That trauma was a nearly fatal perforated uterus leading to peritonitis and several painful surgeries all resulting from an intrauterine device. I had not understood that these "birth control devices", widely used in the 1960's, purposely created inflammation in the uterus to prevent pregnancy. Indeed I now consider them an "instrument of the devil" and how they got FDA approval is, in my judgment, a diabolic plot because they have returned to the market recently. I had two small children and a husband who had just joined a busy pediatrics practice when this trauma ensued and I never worked through the residual emotional damage of this very difficult event. After all, modern medical culture gave no credence to any link between the physical and emotional. It was considered weak to recognize emotional wounds. These negative emotions of bitterness and resentment had literally festered into physical disease and somehow I realized, through my vision, that I was being given an opportunity to resolve the cause of my desperate illness. I would eventually come to understand that any miracle healing had to begin at the cause or origin of the "dis-ease". Frankly, this realization serves as a primary motivator for my writing this book.

For decades, I had pushed back the unresolved emotional pain from that trauma by becoming a workaholic. I had not forgiven people whom I had trusted but whom I felt had failed me nearly costing me my life. It's right there in God's Word that forgiving is a pre-requisite for healing, but I had no idea I was "cancering myself" all those years through unresolved soul wounds. My religion had never taught me to cast my cares on God and I never knew it was sinful to hold a grudge regardless of circumstances. In fact I had no idea that sin is actually breaking both natural and spiritual law and our body-minds inevitably suffer from it. Neither did I grasp the reality of the Holy Spirit. I knew that words could really hurt emotionally, but did not realize they could impact physical health. I honestly lived 40 years in my own wilderness believing that, as a nice Christian person, I should "suck it up" and not bother God or anyone else with my problems. I had copious toxins stored up to burn away in that vision. These toxins were, as the vision revealed, the origin of my cancer. It was no wonder the cancer had returned - particularly in light of the incidents of emotional and physical trauma that occurred within the six months before that return.

After envisioning this poison boiling away, I immediately felt considerably less helpless and much stronger in the faith that I would have victory over this tumor. The first return visit to church was Sunday after the oil service. Yet the enemy, our accuser, well knows the power of words and thoughts so that, by that time, my peace was very much disturbed by conflicting thoughts. Sitting ten feet from where I'd felt lifted off the floor just three days previously, I was overwhelmed with doubts and mental accusations: "What makes you think you deserve to be healed when so many better people than you die of cancer every day?" "The tumor is still there so you didn't get your miracle."

Tag Team "Angels" Save the Day

In the depth of my pre-service despair, God sent me another human "angel" as someone tapped on my shoulder from the row behind. I turned to see a beautiful young woman with the most engagingly warm expression saying, "You have been on my heart since Wednesday night and I feel I need to pray for you. Would you mind telling me a little more about your illness?" I heard myself blurt out my inner conflict, and, instantly, she became a gentle teacher of God's Word regarding healing. After the service, she spent considerable time walking me through a great deal of Healing Scripture in a sensitive and empowering way. She erased all my doubts about God's will regarding healing, indeed my healing. She literally handed me "the sword of the Spirit" so I could stand and fight. She never pushed herself into my life or gossiped about our conversations, but I know she prayed fervently and Biblically for me throughout my ordeal. What a Godsend! I have since learned that she is actually a Physician's Assistant so she understood, but was not swayed by, my dire diagnosis while she encouraged me so tirelessly. Thank God for putting me "on her heart". What she taught me is woven throughout the rest of this book. She carried truth, itself, in her demeanor and words. The powerful Healing Scriptures I refer to are available both in Appendix One of this book and in text and audio on my blog: www.realhealthhope.com.

A week later, I had a CT guided needle biopsy showing only "fatty and fibrous tissue" but the diagnosing doctors just shook their heads and said, "We aren't convinced; and it is still not operable". Something stirred in my spirit for several days, and I heard myself tell my husband, "I'm going to your alma mater (which is a top ten medical center about 150 miles from our home) for a second opinion." I fully encourage anyone dealing with any disease to get more than one opinion before making any treatment decisions. I also encourage all to pray persistently BEFORE deciding on a course of action. Please listen to your spirit stirring and choose only what you are fully at peace to do. So many people hear the "C word", jump into the first thing suggested, and, then pray or put themselves on prayer lists "for good measure". If you get nothing else from this book, I implore you to reverse that order. Your medical records are legally your property and you can get a copy of them, including digital copies of scans, to use in obtaining additional opinions. Don't worry about offending doctors. They are used to people getting second opinions. Whatever you do, do it in response to dialogue with God - out of faith and not out of fear.

I am compelled to admit, I am not sure it was God's will for me to have surgery because I was still such a prayer novice that I didn't make my decision after dialogue with God. I just reacted to a stirring in my spirit and that could have been my own spirit or even the enemy prodding me. It has since occurred to me that I may have rushed that decision in a moment of panic. God stuck with me throughout the terribly difficult surgery experience; yet, had I known then what I know now about prayer, the surgery may well not have been necessary. God only knows for certain.

Priority Authority Is A Must

Prayer focus is so important that I am compelled to break from my own story right here and share a practical excerpt from Dr. David Younggi Cho's, book, *The Fourth Dimension VOL I*. The authority we must give priority to in making our decisions is God, and we do that by learning to pray for His guidance BEFORE making health decisions. I preface the following prayer directive saying that, if you feel you are weak in personal faith, ask God for your full measure of faith because it is the currency of heaven. You will benefit, also, from the prayer agreement of a mature believing Christian as Scripture says in Matthew 18:19, *Again I tell you, if two of you on earth agree (harmonize together, make a symphony together) about whatever [anything and everything] they may ask, it will come to pass and be done for them by My Father in heaven.*

Dr. Cho's prayer directive:

"God will never bring about any of His great works without coming through your own personal faith. It is taken for granted that you have faith, for the Bible says that God has dealt to each and every one of us a measure of faith. You have faith whether you feel it or not. There are, however, certain ways your faith works and links you to the Heavenly Father who dwells within you." [4]

The Bible teaches:

"Faith is the substance of things hoped for." (Hebrews 11:1)

"Faith comes by hearing and hearing by the Word of God." (Romans 10:17)

The Greek for "word" in Romans 10 is not "logos" (written word) but "Rhema" (spoken word). Faith specifically comes by hearing the spoken or saying word of God. That is a specific word to a specific person in a specific situation. You are expecting God to put His spoken word into your own spirit to direct your choices. Dr. Cho teaches us how to get our Rhema.

First, Cho counsels you to put yourself in neutral gear - not "drive" or "reverse" and pray, "Lord I am here and I will listen to your voice. I will go if you say go and I am not going if you say no." [5] Ask God your specific question that you have in your heart such as: "Should I get a second medical opinion?" "Should I choose the treatment path Dr. _____ has suggested?" "If I choose to not have surgery or _____, what should I do? "Is there something blocking manifestation of my healing? If so, what do I need to do to remove it?"

Second, ask God to reveal HIS will through your own desire. In other words, ask God to compel you to want what he wants for you or to intend to do what He intends for you to do. [6] It is Scriptural to do so as it states in the following passages:

Delight yourself also in the Lord, and He will give you the desires and secret petitions of your heart. (Psalms 37:4, AMP)

Whatever you ask for in prayer, believe that you have received it, and it will be yours... and when you stand praying, if you hold anything against anyone, forgive him, so that your Father in heaven may forgive you your sins." (Mark 11:24-25, NIV)

For it is God who works in you, both to will and to act according to His good purpose. (Philippians 2:13, NIV)

Third, pray through as described above and wait upon the Lord until God gives you divine desire. Do not be in a hurry to jump up and say, "I've got it." Satan and your own spirit (soul or will) can also give desires. Time is always a test. Wait patiently and your own desire and satan's will become increasingly weaker but the desire from Holy Spirit becomes stronger and stronger. Wait and receive the divine desire. God knows the ideal schedule. [7]

Fourth, screen that desire through Holy Scripture. If you pray against the written word of God, satan will speak a counterfeit message. Holy Spirit will never contradict God's Word (logos). If you don't have the confidence to do this, go to your minister, pastor, or a mature spiritual mentor for confirmation. Ask them for Scriptures to guide you. (I would add, be absolutely certain your "mentor" has full faith in God's will for your healing to manifest. Avoid anyone who says anything doubting God's will to have you fully restored to health because that is man's doctrine and not God's. Keep the energy positive. [8]

Fifth, ask God for a beckoning signal from your circumstances. If God truly has spoken to your heart, then He is bound to give you a signal from the outside external world. Ask for such a sign like Elijah and Gideon did in the Bible. (1 Kings 17 and Judges 6:17) [9]

Finally, pray to know God's timing. Pray until you have real peace without any restlessness of spirit. You will have the God kind of faith that is the original Greek language in Mark 11:22-23 and you will be within God's timing. Spend time meditating in God's written word so He will have material to work with in you. Ask Him for Scriptures to help you understand the decisions you are praying for guidance in. Ask and then get quiet in your entire being and listen. He will speak to your soul. [10]

This is not a formula prayer. It is a Biblical approach to prayer asking for a Rhema (saying) Word from God.

Again, I strongly encourage you to take time and earnestly seek divine guidance BEFORE making treatment decisions rather than hurrying to make a decision rooted in fear and then asking people to pray that your decisions work out. The latter is futile much like sitting down to a meal you know is terribly unhealthy and asking God to "bless it to your nourishment" anyway. God will not go against His own Word or His laws of Creation even though, being sovereign, He could. Doing so would begat chaos. (See Psalms 139:2 in Young's Literal Translation.)

Miracles, Music and Heavenly Messengers Converge

Returning to my own story, I did eventually go to my husband's alma mater for the second opinion, and a brilliant surgeon there deemed the tumor "operable" which, at the time, I considered miraculous. That pronouncement notwithstanding, the anticipated four hour operation became nine difficult hours. In fact, God stepped in several times. Remember that troublesome tumor in my superior mesenteric vein (SMV) I referred to earlier - the one the surgeons in my "strike one surgery" said they completely plucked from the vein just five days after my first pancreatic tumor was removed?

This time a vein graft actually was required which meant the SMV had to be clamped off for the process. I'm told that clamp off has about a fifteen minute time limit which is why a graft is harvested from another part of the body before the diseased vein is clamped and cut. Talk about a miracle, my SMV was clamped off for nearly four hours and all but one of my potential donor veins were wasted in failed efforts. The surgeons had warned my family that they were running out of options before they made the last grafting effort. Miraculously, the last graft held. We have tremendous healing faculties built into our wonderfully made bodies. Supplemental vein generation is one of those mechanisms. My body had likely generated some alternative vein capacity while the SMV tumor was forming. This vein generation mechanism also created new vein routes to replace all three harvested grafts. Countless healing miracles are ever present in our wonderfully created bodies.

By the time the final vein graft held, my abdomen had been through nine hours of difficult surgery and surgeons could not close me so I was strapped together and kept unconscious for five days. I have no recollection of time passing while in that induced coma except a strange sense that I was being ministered to. Prayer energy buoyed me positively and sometimes I sensed I was back at Pastor Tom's church where I had my oil service. The folks of strong faith in that church, were interceding in prayer for me as were other strong believers and I was somehow aware of that prayer energy. When I awakened and my husband told me I'd been unconscious five days, I couldn't believe it.

For the entire three-week hospitalization, whenever I was asleep or unconscious, the words of Handel's "Messiah" (taken from Isaiah 9:6) played through my spirit.

> For unto us a child is born, unto us a son is given:
> and the government shall be upon his shoulder:
> and his name shall be called Wonderful, Counselor,
> The mighty God, The everlasting Father, The Prince of Peace.

Even now, when I hear that profound music, a certain indescribable sensation comes over me. I've since learned why this particular music is so Spiritually profound and it illustrates, to me, the timeless love of this God that Isaiah and Handel could not describe with a single name. In his book, *Spiritual Lives of the Great Composers,* Patrick Kavanaugh writes, "Handel's (personal) servant has become frustrated because, for days he has prepared and served Handel untouched trays of food . . . Once again, he steels himself to go through the same routine, muttering under his breath about how oddly temperamental musicians can be. As he swings open the door to the composer's room, the servant stops in his tracks. The startled composer, tears streaming down his face, turns to his servant and cries out, 'I did think I did see all heaven before me, and the great God Himself.' George Frederic Handel had just finished writing a movement that would take its place in history as the 'Hallelujah Chorus'."[11]

I hope my readers can grasp the significance to me of that music being there for me while I was in a physical and mental, but **not spiritual** coma. Our God is creative - in every way all the time. Surgeon Bernie Siegel says, "Music opens up a spiritual window." He kept it playing in his operating rooms.[12]

During my unconscious time while Handel's music played in my spirit, my family kept a waiting room vigil. My son's wife was due to deliver their first child, but she unselfishly insisted my son come be with his dad and sister until I woke up. One time my daughter visited my ICU bedside and actually saw my angel of light hovering at the head of my bed. When I was stabilized enough for her to return home, her young son, who had not been told of his mother's encounter, showed her a remarkably accurate drawing of my angel. To me, this is more evidence of interaction between heaven and earth beginning with powerful prayer that calls in ministering angels. I felt that prayer energy - believers' prayer is powerful focused energy. During both my "strike one" and "strike two" hospitalizations, my family's presence brought palpable sustaining energy. They were faithful.

The "strike two" hospital saga was a long process including a difficult bout with infection that required hospital staff to don HAZMAT gear when entering my room. Additionally, it took me a while to adjust to losing half my stomach, pyloric valve, several inches of small colon, and gall bladder along with another one third of my pancreas. The doctors avoided eye contact when they talked about "spots" on the pancreas remnant, liver and lungs. Strangely, I felt as though I was on a different wavelength than the doctors and never participated in the subtle negativity of their body language. Once out of quarantine, I just asked them what I had to do to be discharged. They said, "hold down food 24 hours and be able to walk around the nurses' station with a walker". It was like a stop action movie in the hallway when I pulled that one off because staff knew I could barely make it to the bathroom six feet from the bed. My altered digestive system anatomy suddenly quieted. I found myself pushing that walker like plowing fertile ground while jaws dropped and cheers went up. I won my "get out of jail free card" on Christmas Eve. Surely my angel participated in that event.

Home for Christmas

We made the four-hour road trip home in driving rain late on Christmas Eve. I was probably released a bit before I was ready, but I think the doctors wanted me to be home for what they feared might be my last Christmas. I remember the sweat suit I wore had fit well upon admission to the hospital, but was several sizes too large on this trip home. My husband practically carried me up the three steps into our house and I fell into bed in that darn sweat suit because I had no strength to change clothes. But I was "home free" ... or so I thought. I was a veteran at recovering from difficult surgery even though this one was the daddy of them all. "Strike Two" seemed to be over, but it had been a "foul tip" and I had to stand in the box for another pitch.

The vascular surgeon who had been called in for the last ditch vein graft had insisted I take a blood thinning drug to keep pressure off the graft. I needed a local doctor to oversee dosage yet I hadn't established a primary physician after withdrawing from the state university medical center after the "sorry about your luck" diagnosis. Our daughter called a surgeon friend who very kindly helped us get set up with a regional hospital lab to monitor the blood thinner before he left town on holiday. My husband and I literally dragged my body to that lab every other day for blood tests.

Several days into that process, I bled profusely from the bowel and barely made it to the emergency room in time. After many transfusions, I was scanned upwards and downwards never finding the bleeding source although doctors felt it was surely linked to the blood thinning pharmaceutical. I was air lifted back to my husband's alma mater. It was another miracle that the bleeding miraculously stopped without further intervention. I never took the blood-thinning drug again although I do take a natural blood thinner daily - garlic. I've never had another issue.

Later it occurred to me that a miraculous beneficial result of this "bleed out" was a thorough clearing out of the copious residual pharmaceuticals I had in my system from the extended surgery, induced coma etc. As always, God was able to use an evil ploy of the enemy for good (see Romans 8:28) and it literally sped up my emotional and mental recovery, which enabled me to expedite the "be my own doctor" program sooner.

The Perfect Coach Gives Perfect Signals

By the time I returned home yet again, I looked and felt like an army had marched over my body and I needed a survival plan. It felt like a late inning "at bat" and I had used up my "strike one" and now "strike two" so it was "home run or else". I realized I needed to work with my Creator, the Great Physician, Father God rather than putting all my faith into secular medicine.

Father God, my "batting coach", was sending "perfect signals" all the way - the ultimate one being His early morning assurance, "The Bible is true", shared earlier. The love and encouragement He poured forth was personalized and critical. I began to crave everything about this amazing Lord. I had a lot of dead time to make up for - not because I feared dying but because I developed a strong desire to become a fruitful "believing believer" rather than a nominal Christian. I'd glimpsed love and promises beyond anything I could have ever asked or imagined. I'd discovered a full bank account of grace I had never known existed. I wanted to live to investigate and share this blessed inheritance. I heard myself praying continuously that I might get through this ordeal and become an encourager to others. I was moving toward the light rather than away from the darkness—a direction that is naturally and supernaturally energizing.

Please understand that I have not shared my story to make this book about me but to let my readers know that I write from a platform of experience. I want to offer my readers real hope. Hoping is NOT wishing. Hoping is expecting, intending for good things to happen and boldly saying so. Hope is also realizing that healing is part of our heavenly inheritance. We need to raise our expectations high enough to reach into heaven and pull down the promise of healing.

That promise is part of our "Kingdom inheritance". As Pastor Bill Johnson often says: "You can have a million dollars in a bank account and starve to death if you don't know what you have." [13] Ephesians 3:20 provides one of many passages I believe illustrates how short our expectations often fall: *Now to him who is able to do immeasurably more than all we ask or imagine, according to his power that is at work within us...* (NIV).

We have a God who cares for our bodies; the bodies He created. In this creation, our identities are not our bodies but we can **only** fulfill the exciting and meaningful plans God has for us in *"His Kingdom coming on earth as in heaven"* if we steward our bodies for health. (Matthew 6 and Luke 11).

God tells us in Jeremiah 29:11-13:

> *"For I know the plans I have for you,' declares the LORD, "plans to prosper you and not to harm you, plans to give you hope and a future. Then you will call upon me and come and pray to me, and I will listen to you. You will seek me and find me when you seek me with all your heart."* (NIV)

three

Embracing The Power of Love

During my fight to overcome the medical diagnosis and live in the beauty of a new life - whole, complete and healthy – I entered into the power of a love that **changes everything**. A most surprising revelation to me was a moment in prayer that I realized I did not want the prayer time to ever end. I had "habits" from my years as a workaholic and one of them was moving from task to task somewhat compulsively. Per my old habit, I too often divided focus between prayer and what I "planned to do next". God yearns for our total focus just as any loving parent yearns for intimate time with their child. We want our children and grandchildren to **voluntarily** put down the cell phone and focus on our conversation. I sensed the height and depth of God's love when I became aware that I actually did want **everything changed** and was no longer holding back "sacred cows" nor tempted to cut my prayer time short and "get back to life". God is a wonderful conversationalist when we are **totally present** with Him.

As my time spent in God's Word increased, my prayer matured to include my visceral gratitude for each new connection in my "dot-to-dot miracle". Then, I found myself praying that I might live to become an encourager to others because I was learning so much I wanted to share. The desperate souls I met in oncology waiting rooms had grabbed my heart and I felt real compassion rather than old familiar sympathy. I realized I loved people whom I didn't even know. I knew their plight first hand. I became strongly compelled to share what I was learning in my own trip through *"the valley of the shadow of death"* (Psalms 23:4). I found myself praying for other individuals in those waiting room - sometimes carrying little "Healing Scripture" books with me to give away or leave on tables.

The power of love only changes **all things** when we surrender **all things** Reversing the impact of cancer and locking cancer out of our lives can be done. In choosing life and real health, we end up living a beautiful life – spiritually, emotionally and physically. We end up living in the power of love, governed by the laws, or principles of love. In the process of choosing health, we enter into alignment with these principles of love that lead to health and are compelled to make certain changes in our lifestyles. Intentional changes lead to a richer life than we can imagine. Intentional changes lead to living in the presence of God's love and entering into His kingdom of heaven (where there is no disease) while still walking on earth. Jesus said; . . . *neither shall they say, Lo, here! or, There! for lo, the kingdom of God is within you.* Luke 17:21 (ASV)

Pure Laws of Love

Let's examine three basic categories where natural and super-natural laws of love converge as we seek to understand all we have available to enable us to lock cancer out of our lives. Nineteenth century scientist-theologian, Henry Drummond, implied in his classic, *Natural Law and the Spiritual World*[1] *that* the term "law" essentially means "a series of linked phenomena" responsible for explaining order that has already been set in place or created. Law is law - it is in place where we "see" it in nature and "know" it in spirit without conflict. Jesus used parables of natural law to illustrate spiritual law - for example, the parable of the sower. Drummond actually says natural and spiritual laws exist as "the same law". I believe we can apply Drummond's insights to the "cascade of events" that can move us from the "healthy state" to the "disease state" which I refer to later and list more specifically in Appendix Five. The reversal back to the "healthy state" has both natural and spiritual aspects, which are within the "pure laws (principles) of health" in love, work, and stewardship.

Galatians 5:22-23 I believe, can help us understand Drummond's point regarding "laws" or principles underpinning health: *And the fruit of the Spirit is: Love, joy, peace, long-suffering, kindness, goodness, faith, meekness, temperance: **against such there is no law**.* (YLT) "Long-suffering" can also be translated as "patience" in this Scripture.

Simply stated, the price to pay for real health and wholeness is living a beautiful life spiritually, emotionally, mentally, and physically.

Whenever I say this in a seminar, I sometimes sense a "bristling" within some attendees who have lost loved ones to cancer - loved ones they believe "lived beautiful lives". I understand the sensitivity and I mean to speak about this subject compassionately, but I cannot hold back insights that may help keep other loved ones from being lost too early. "The good die young" is a cliché rooted in a grieving need to explain away losses such as those cancer too often causes. Somehow, our thoughts and words bubble up from broken hearts where the enemy has painted an evil bulls eye and buried his lying fiery darts such as, "We can't know God's purpose in these things." Or, "Sometimes God chooses not to heal 'for the greater glory," etc.

In fact, many churches and denominations build un-Biblical doctrines to rationalize sorrowful disappointment. The enemy gets his licks in when false doctrines knock the "Sword of the Spirit" out of the hands of God's people, dilute their prayers, and empower the "thief who *comes to steal, kill, and destroy"* (see John 10:10). We will continue looking at these difficult subjects because we often mourn the loss of righteous loved ones to disease like cancer not realizing that what they may have thought or spoken into their own lives ultimately undermined their health. Please bear with me on this point for now. I understand that it is sensitive; however, I believe our next topic will begin to bring some soothing insights.

Three "Pure Laws" of Peace and Health

The words we speak to ourselves are powerful. *The power of life and death are in the tongue* (Proverbs 18:21). The power to achieve peace and health lies within each of us. In fact, there are three pure laws of peace and health noted within Scripture. They are love, work and stewardship. Love includes forgiveness – a process that cleanses spiritual toxins from our minds and bodies. Work includes keeping our reason for living before us and focusing on the purpose we have yet to fulfill on earth. And stewardship encompasses loving ourselves enough to do what we need to do to lock the door of our lives against cancer.

LOVE:

When Jesus was asked what the most important commandment was, He replied in Luke 10:27: *You must love the Lord your God with all your heart and with all your soul and with all your strength and with all your mind; and your neighbor as yourself.*

That commandment means forgive, bless, do good, pray for, laugh with, worship with . . . and, did I mention, **FORGIVE!**

WORK:

Work is not part of the curse resulting from original sin but is part of the original blessing [2] as noted in Genesis 2:15: *And the Lord God took the man and put him in the Garden of Eden to tend and guard and keep it.*

Everyone has a purpose in the grand scheme of things and that purpose will include productive work, whether in an avocation, or a vocation approached with enthusiasm and excellence. We are created to be creative and fruitful.

STEWARDSHIP:

"YOU" are not your body but you have one to steward which includes managing food, water, breathing habits, sleep habits, play habits, words spoken and written, thoughts, sights, sounds, emotions - all of which impact every single life process. The Apostle Paul told the Corinthians in 1 Corinthians 6:19: *Do you not know that your body is the temple (the very sanctuary) of the Holy Spirit Who lives within you, Whom you have received [as a Gift] from God? You are not your own.*

Stewardship is really taking back dominion within your mind and body from the enemy. Jesus paid for the recovery of this dominion on the whipping post and cross. It is in our divine inheritance that we steward by walking it out in our lives.

I am compelled to look at both Scripture and science relative to each of these "pure laws" in order to establish insights that enrich our discussion moving into chapters focusing specifically on how to do life in a way that not only slams the cancer door but flings wide open the health door.

What Has Love to Do with Living in the "Healthy State"?

God is Love

Love is *who* God IS. I would add that Love is HOW God is. God created human beings because He is love and love needs a target. God wanted a family as Frank Viola so eloquently explains in his book, *From Eternity to Here*. Viola ends his introduction promising "a staggering look at the ageless purpose that drives your God. For that purpose is the very reason you exist."[3] God wanted a family made in His image who could love Him back but He did not want puppets who had no choice but to love Him. Rather He wanted kids who would see His unconditional love for them and join into a loving relationship that is the very antithesis of guilt driven "religion". God's love is healing – not condemning.

When we begin to realize that God loves us and created us to be loved, we begin to love God in return. If we love Him back, we live with Him in heavenly places and our entire perspective is unworldly because we count on His promises and we draw on our divine inheritance. It's a "view from the throne" and it is pure joy because, while our bodies "live with our feet on earth", our souls (mind, will, emotions) can actually hover above the fray. By that I mean we can choose NOT to become insulted, offended or wounded by what those around us say and do - those who operate from a worldly perspective, which too often gets them in situations that wound their own souls. Their offensive words and actions towards us most often have roots in their own soul wounds.

Loving Others

Remembering that "The Bible is True", let's look at some Scripture. Jesus brought a clear "love message" which may seem unfair by worldly standards; however, He, of course, had full knowledge of the science that converged with His teaching because He was there at the creation of it. Let's recall the love lesson in Luke 10:25-28:

> And then a certain lawyer arose to try (test, tempt) Him (Jesus), saying, Teacher, what am I to do to inherit everlasting life [that is, to partake of eternal salvation in the Messiah's kingdom]?
> Jesus said to him, What is written in the Law? How do you read it?
> And he replied, You must love the Lord your God with all your heart and with all your soul and with all your strength and with all your mind; and your neighbor as yourself.
> And Jesus said to him, You have answered correctly; do this, and you will live [enjoy active, blessed, endless life in the kingdom of God].

When the lawyer's follow up question was, *"and who is my neighbor?"*, Jesus told the familiar parable of the Good Samaritan in which a Jewish man lay beaten and bleeding on the side of the road. A Samaritan (traditionally hostile to Jews) came to the injured man, stopped and cared for the victim even helping him to an inn and paying for his lodging while he healed. (See Luke 10.)

The lesson, of course, is that everyone is our neighbor and "the law of love" means we even love and help our enemies. On another occasion, Jesus taught: *Love your enemies, bless those cursing you, do good to those hating you, and pray for those accusing you falsely, and persecuting you.* (Matthew 5:44, YLT)

Tough assignment? Perhaps, but it is unimaginably empowering to do so. Jesus modeled His instructions. Perhaps you answer, "yes, but Jesus was God so He could do things we mere mortals should not be expected to do". I used to think so too, but, in truth, Jesus was fully man (see Hebrews 2:17 and Philippians 2:7) who (by strength gained in prayerful relationship with the Father) lived without sin because, as He explained in John 5:19: *He only did what He saw the Father do.*

He had to live out His life fully human so that He could be the legal ultimate "stand in" sacrifice (the "spotless lamb") for all other fully human beings and, thereby, restore dominion that another fully human being, Adam, lost through disobedience. British minister Graham Cooke's insight regarding this restoration is profound: "If satan had known what Jesus would accomplish in His crucifixion and resurrection, he would have killed everyone who was trying to kill Jesus." Why? It is because the cross was a successful stealth move to restore God's dominion on earth and, basically, to exchange "Karma" (You get what you deserve.) for "Grace" (You get what you could never deserve). Galatians 3:13 succinctly states, *"Christ redeemed us from the curse of the law by becoming a curse for us, for it is written: 'Cursed is everyone who is hung on a tree'."* Sickness was part of the curse in Deuteronomy but Jesus reversed it and restored Kingdom dominion.

The man, Jesus, is alive, glorified and seated at the right hand of God intervening and advocating for those who accept Him. His followers cannot visit where He is buried like the followers of mortal religious leaders, but we can join Him in His throne room and actually live from that perspective right now. I am not suggesting that we are required to live a perfect life in order to have our healing manifest. The finished work of Jesus covers us with amazing grace. We could never deserve it. Does that grace give us a license to purposely sin? Of course not, but the blood on that cross covers us if we do slip up and we are sincerely repentant. God is not mad at us or out to get us. My own story illustrates this. He IS love.

I practically ignored Him for decades but He never gave up on me and I'm no more special to Him than any other human being. He's *"no respecter of persons"* (Acts 10:34). He has no favorites.

If this is news to you, you can bring yourself up to speed by reading and meditating on the four gospels (especially John) and the epistles (especially Romans without breaking between chapters 7 and 8 and Colossians) in the New Testament. Biblical meditation is empowering in limitless ways. Biblical meditation means **filling our minds** with truth unlike other forms of meditation that aim at **emptying our minds**. Empty minds can be fertile ground for the enemy of our souls to plant unhealthy seeds. Think of it this way, Jesus was "the Word made flesh" and that same powerful, living Word becomes part of our own flesh as we meditate upon it. I know this is true from personal experience and it makes sense in light of quantum mechanics because the matter (elemental substance) in our bodies is in constant vibration as are spoken words. We all yearn to vibrate with the very rhythm of God's life force.

Bono, lead singer of the group U2, showed surprisingly deep Christian insight during an interview with Frank Viola (co-author of the profound book, *Jesus* Manifesto). Bono's revealing comments pave the way for understanding how to live in the rhythm of God's life force as he said:

"My understanding of the Scriptures has been made simple by the person of Christ. Christ teaching that God is love . . . God IS love, and as much as I respond in allowing myself to be transformed by that love and acting in that love, that's my religion . . . It's a mind-blowing concept that the God who created the universe might be looking for company, a real relationship with people . . ." [4]

Bono also talked about the difference between Karma and Grace and why Grace trumps Karma which leads me to ask: Who could disagree that every one on earth would be happier if **we only had to deal with other people who** "allowed themselves to be transformed", as Bono said, by this "love teaching" of Jesus? On the other hand, **what's actually in it for us to be the ones treating others lovingly**? I can think of two things immediately– joy and health– actually, three things because there is enormous power in truly loving the unlovely. Stay with me; I believe you'll see how this can work for you.

Can we really change our environment, our relationships or our own health by loving those who hurt and offend us? Yes! We can and we must because such living follows both scientific and Kingdom or spiritual law. I'm talking about much more than "the law of attraction". I'm talking about "Let there be peace on earth and let it begin with me." [5] Can the message in the words of one popular song actually impact whether we live in the "disease state" or the "healthy state"? The answer must be yes because a "pure law of the universe" says so. Who could live in a world without love? Receiving it is great– giving it is even greater because it exponentially multiplies that love. It's the same principle as sowing seed.

Loving Yourself

We often gloss over the "as yourself" in the earlier quoted Luke 10 Scripture, but it is critical to our health that we "love ourselves". We cannot love others "as ourselves" if we do not first love ourselves. Earlier I shared the erroneous doctrine I developed in my youth from a perversion of the teaching, "I am third". Obviously this perversion is a counterfeit of Jesus' words from Luke 10:27, *You must love the Lord your God with all your heart and with all your soul and with all your strength and with all your mind; and your neighbor as yourself.*

God first, others second, then self third is the perversion; and, like all the enemy's ploys, it "seems" good to man (me). The truth is that if you love the Lord with all your heart, soul, strength, and mind", you won't be able to keep yourself from loving either others or loving yourself. You must love God and others "as your REAL self"– "that self" whom The Lord loves, values, and *"has plans to prosper and not harm"* (Jeremiah 29:11). That would be the same "self" who sees himself or herself through the eyes of Jesus and The Father– through the very eyes of LOVE itself. According to Pastor Kris Vallotton, "Calling it humility when not loving yourself is still thinking about yourself. If you malign your own soul, you undermine health and prosperity. Not loving yourself is disagreeing with God." [6]

Jesus made it clear how He differed from the enemy of our souls when He said per John 10:10: *The thief comes only in order to steal and kill and destroy. I came that they may have and enjoy life, and have it in abundance (to the full, till it overflows).*

I hope you meditate on this passage until it is part of your very being so you know how important you are to God. I do not apologize for repeating it because it must become part of our flesh if we want to be "in health".

In more arguably scientific resources, I have also read of ways we "cancer ourselves". Dr. David Servan-Schreiber, M.D., PhD, best explains this dynamic in his discussion of a "C" type personality ("C" for cancer). The essentials include, "People who, rightly or wrongly, never felt fully welcome in their childhood . . . later, to be sure of being loved, they decided to conform to the best of their ability to what was expected of them rather than follow their own desires . . . Rarely angry (sometimes never), they become 'really nice people' . . . They avoid conflict." [7] He further explains that the common denominator most observed is 'the feeling of helplessness' which has been much studied as a root of disease and a block to healing.

I'm compelled to wonder how many of our loved ones who have succumbed to cancer lived what they and others thought were "beautiful lives" even though they were really walking in the self deprecating and diabolical parameters of a "C" type personality neither fully realizing that they were who God's Word says they are nor that God is who He says He is.

We need not feel helpless because our souls are wounded by past trauma, sin (either our own or sin against us), or by being chronically offended without dealing with the toxins of that offense. I will soon share some amazing and practical revelation on soul healing. The good news is that if we can "cancer ourselves", then we can certainly "un-cancer ourselves".

What Has Work to Do with Living in the "Healthy State"?

Dr. Albert Schweitzer always believed that the best medicine for any illness he might have was the knowledge that he had a job to do plus a good sense of humor. [8]

God is a perpetually creative being and it follows that we who are created in His image are creative beings as well. He is Spirit and our "selves" are spirit also. Surely it also follows that we cannot be fully whole either physically, mentally, or spiritually if we are not creatively living and working productively per our individual design. Creating is work and work is creating. Each of us has abilities, gifts, talents, passions and attributes we must use either vocationally or avocationally in order to "satisfy" our inborn natures. Every person has a purpose in the grand scheme of things and that purpose must include productive work approached with enthusiasm and excellence. Our work, then, is meant to be done "unto God". After all, He tells us: *Beloved, I pray that you may prosper in every way and [that your body] may keep well, even as [I know] your soul keeps well and prospers.* (3 John 1:2, AMP)

There is a great difference between "punching the time clock just to get a paycheck" and "joyfully working unto God according to our unique inborn design". When we work "unto God", we know He will appreciate it even if we may feel that others don't. He is a proud parent when we do our best whatever the task. Am I saying that every person is likely to hold a job that automatically thrills him or her every minute of every day? Hardly! Yet, whether it is in formal employment or in a volunteer position, a person physically, mentally, and emotionally needs to use their God given talents creating goods or providing services in a way that satisfies their innate purpose and vents their wholesome passion.

Certainly, "on the job attitude" is critical and there can be no drudgery unless we let the enemy convince us our work is meaningless and unproductive. If we entertain feeling helpless and stuck either in unemployment or in an employment situation that does not fit our individual aptitudes, our health is at risk. The Apostle Paul taught in Colossians 3:17: . . . *whatever ye may do in word or in work, do all things in the name of the Lord Jesus– giving thanks to the God and Father, through him.* (YLT)

Further, we can learn much from the 16th century monk, Brother Lawrence, who spent every day in the drudgery of medieval monastery kitchen duty yet maintained constant joyful communication with the Lord. [9]

Another great lesson in the sanctity of work lies in the life of the Apostle Paul who labored as a tentmaker to support himself while traveling all over the known first century world preaching the gospel of the Lord. I recently heard Pastor Bill Johnson point out how God's value for honest toil is illustrated by the fact that even remnants of Paul's **work clothes** were powerfully anointed,[10] *So that handkerchiefs or towels or aprons which had touched his skin (while he toiled at manual labor) were carried away and put upon the sick, and their diseases left them and the evil spirits came out of them.* (Acts 19:12, AMP)

Dr. Bernie Siegel's book, *Love, Medicine and Miracles: Lessons Learned about Self Healing from a Surgeon's Exceptional Patients* helps us understand the beautiful life that we are invited into: "When we awaken to our mortality, we refuse to live the life that is killing us and start living and being our true selves. On a practical level it may mean changing occupations, moving, healing or ending relationships and bringing meaning and a new attitude into life and working for the right Lord. Your life is stored in your body. Neither people nor body cells do well living off someone else's production– doing so maligns a person's identity as a unique and important creation. Remember that "malign" is the root work for "malignancy".

Christ's . . . message is this: If you do not bring forth what is within you, what you do not bring forth will destroy you. If you bring forth what is within you, what you do bring forth will save you.' He (Jesus) is talking about our feelings and body memories." [11]

Dr. Siegel, whose career included many patients diagnosed with diseases like cancer, further observes: "Survivors take time to be still and listen. Take time to be still and **listen** to the voice within you and the voice which will come to you . . . If you **listen**, you will **learn your purpose here** and be able to die joyfully, knowing that you have served in your way and fulfilled the reasons for your creation." [12]

Of course Dr. Siegel means, "die joyfully" when your earthly "assignment" is completed and you are satisfied rather than "die joyfully from the disease you might currently battle". We are meant to live out our lives and die satisfied. It is a lie of the enemy that we must all die of a disease. God's Word and, therefore, His will never dooms us to disease because disease is not from God. "The Lord's Prayer" states it clearly in (Matthew 6:10): *Your Kingdom come, Your will be done on earth as in it is in heaven.*

There is no disease in heaven. Thus, according to His Word in this prayer, God means for there to be no sickness on earth. Psalms 91 also reassures us of God's intention so that we may line our own intent up with His: *He shall call upon Me, and I will answer him; I will be with him in trouble, I will deliver him and honor him. With long life will I satisfy him and show him My salvation.* (Psalms 91:15-16, AMP)

Throughout the book, *Overcoming Blocks to Healing,* Bill Banks, who was miraculously healed of cancer, shares stories of healthy elderly believers who, satisfied their assignment was completed, peacefully slipped out of this life.

I encourage you to consider the advice of Dr. Bernie Siegel as well as that earlier shared from Dr. David Younggi Cho in seeking the Rhema Word of God specifically for your personal situation whether it is treatment decisions or life changes that will bring you into health. Every miracle is interactive beginning with dialoguing with God even if it's a foxhole prayer like mine.

Stewardship of The Body is a Tremendous Opportunity

In the "pure laws of health" just discussed– Love, Work, and Stewardship, the first two may seem more ethereal than the latter because so many anti-cancer books concentrate largely on very rigid regimens of nutrition, exercise, detoxification, etc. in more of a one protocol fits all perspective than I could be comfortable with. Furthermore, many "spiritual resources" dance around mentioning God in an effort to walk the "universalism" line. Universalism is so inclusive of a wide variety of beliefs about who Jesus is, that it fails to consider Christ as the only true God whose blood shed on the cross is sufficient for healing our bodies, souls and spirits.

Conversely, I have found few notably spiritual resources that even considered the specifics of stewarding physical health, which may explain what I've observed as the church's lack of concern with disease prevention. I don't mean to offend anyone, but I've been saddened many times to attend a church dinner composed of beautiful dishes containing tremendous quantities of health sabotaging foods such as sugars and hydrogenated fats. The question is whether or not God would go against His own design of our bodies and bless food that interferes with health. Can we turn away from Daniel's dietary lessons and pray God will override unhealthy eating decisions? Stewardship is actively taking back dominion the enemy has subtly chipped away. The serpent basically influenced Eve with a "food commercial" and convinced her and Adam to abandon stewardship responsibilities God had given them.

Mind and Body "In this together"

We will be discussing nutrition, diet, sleep, breathing, and other critical aspects of physical stewardship - indeed body care and maintenance without separating the body from the mind and emotions as most western religious communities unintentionally do and as medical science has been careful to do since 17th century philosopher/mathematician/ scientist Rene` Descartes made a deal with the Pope of his day to "leave the soul (mind/will/emotions) to the "church" so that "medical science would focus only on the body". I found in my research that this agreement still has strong influence in both church and medicine.

Dr. Bruce Lipton, having taught in several medical schools and done considerable research in cellular biology, writes of his own "Cartesian Challenges" saying (regarding his research), "My colleagues almost died of apoplexy at the notion of injecting the body-mind connection into a paper about cell biology . . . My colleagues did not want me to include these implications of my research because the mind is not an acceptable biological concept . . . The mind is a non-localized energy and therefore is not relevant to materialistic biology. Unfortunately, that perception is a 'belief' that has been proven to be patently incorrect in a quantum mechanical universe!" Lipton discusses the "placebo effect" as an illustration then discloses, "The placebo effect is quickly glossed over in medical schools so that students can get to the real *tools* of modern medicine like drugs and surgery . . . This is a major mistake . . . Doctors should let go of their conviction that the body and its parts are essentially stupid and that we need outside intervention to maintain our health." [13]

Because it is Scripturally and biologically sound, we will consider the soul (mind, will, emotions) in our Section Three practical discussion of physical stewardship. I have learned the hard way there are serious consequences in trying to recover health without agreeing with God. We must guard our thought life and train our brain to teach our mouth to **agree with God**." The wise King Solomon wrote in Proverbs 23:7: *For as a man thinks, so is he.*

Rene` Descartes (who is famous for saying "I think, therefore I am.) apparently understood Solomon's point and the Pope of his day did not . . . or perhaps the issue is more one of control than truth? Still Descartes "sold out" regarding the mind-body connection in order to gain papal permission to dissect cadavers and "medical science" followed him down that wrong path for centuries and still resists correcting course. Regardless, the Apostle Paul also agreed with Solomon when he wrote to the Philippians: *Finally, brothers, whatever is true, whatever is noble, whatever is right, whatever is pure, whatever is lovely, whatever is admirable– if anything is excellent or praiseworthy– think about such things.* (Philippians 4:8, NIV)

My point is that "stewardship of our bodies" is ultimately our own responsibility and our **souls cannot be separated from our bodies**. This realization is good news in the face of ever more government maneuvering of the "sick care industry". We have the REAL "health care" tools in our "divine trust fund" and Jesus already activated our inheritance through his death.

Notes:

four

Healing is a Done Deal

He (Jesus) used his servant body to carry our sins to the Cross so we could be rid of sin, free to live the right way. His wounds became your healing. (1 Peter 2:24, MSG)

Time after time, many "believers" are standing in prayer lines and chasing after miracles without perceivably "being healed". As a result, many people steer clear of being "active believers" because, frankly, they are tired of hearing Christians talk about God's healing power while half the members of too many churches are sick even though their names may be on a dozen prayer lists.

Jesus did not keep up with a "prayer list". Even though he had not taken the Roman scourging or bled on the cross yet, in his earthly ministry Jesus did not beg Father God to heal folks. He was a servant and not a beggar. Neither did he dole out sympathy with a long face nor did he ever mention any value or purpose in human suffering. His every action showed us the difference between compassion and sympathy. Bill Johnson expounds on this point best, "Sympathy massages a person within the problem; compassion looks for a way out. Biblical compassion always has the heart of God in mind."[1]

Jesus never said anything sympathetic like, "Well brother, I'd like to see you healed, but we can only pray that the Father's will is done and then hope against hope." He always found a way to change the situation from disease to health. He knew the enemy's power wasn't equal to God's. "God could easily wipe out the whole kingdom of darkness in a moment. God decided it would be more beneficial and more glorious to share His victory with sons and daughters made in His image who can put on display what He's like." [2]

Jesus, teaching us the victorious lifestyle, obviously followed the will of the Father in every way and told us in John 5:19: *So Jesus answered them by saying, I assure you, most solemnly I tell you, the Son is able to do nothing of Himself (of His own accord); but He is able to do only what He sees the Father doing, for whatever the Father does is what the Son does in the same way [in His turn].*

We can understand what is included in our own blood bought inheritance by watching what Jesus does regarding healing the sick. Jesus, a man, was anointed with the Holy Spirit at his baptism in the same way "believers who actually do believe Scripture" have been ever since. Matthew 3:16,17 puts us on the ground at Jesus's baptism:

And having been baptized, Jesus went up immediately from the water, and lo, opened to him were the heavens, and he saw the Spirit of God descending as a dove, and coming upon him, and lo, a voice out of the heavens, saying, 'This is My Son– the Beloved, in whom I did delight. (YLT)

Then, that Holy Spirit led Jesus, as a man, into the wilderness where satan (the enemy of every man's soul) tempted him. It seems satan could not fathom that God would actually send His only son as a human into the domain satan had won by "sweet talking" the first humans. It appears that satan wanted to know who he was up against in this man, Jesus, upon whom the "dove" had just landed; yet, despite satan's goading, Jesus never revealed his divine sonship. Further, in his wilderness trials, Jesus wielded the all-powerful "Sword of the Spirit" or Word of God responding to the enemy's contorting of the same Scripture. Jesus knew God's Word and we must also. It's also important to remember that, in His ministry, Jesus always referred to himself as "son of man". He was not yet the glorified Christ, the Messiah, until after his resurrection. The Apostle Paul in Romans 8:29 called Christ the "first-born among many brethren" and we "believers" who carry "the Sword" are those "many brethren". What a God!

I mention all this to lead to an important point. When we follow Jesus and receive the Holy Spirit, we accept that very same anointing with which Jesus walked out his earthly ministry and **all** that goes with it. What is "**all** that goes with it"? Jesus said it when he came out of the wilderness and went into the temple and read from Isaiah as Luke 4:18 reports: *The Spirit of the Lord is upon me, Because He did anoint me; To proclaim good news to the poor, Sent me to heal the* **broken of heart**, *To proclaim to captives deliverance, And to blind receiving of sight, To send away the bruised with deliverance.* (YLT)

I added emphasis to "broken of heart" because we are about to look further at the importance of having our souls (emotional hearts) healed as a basis for our bodies being healed. We can also observe the reference to body (bruised and blind) and spirit (deliverance from evil spirits). Jesus came to make sure the people of God were sound in body, soul and spirit. Jesus said it plainly and he demonstrated the importance of complete healing throughout his earthly ministry while he was calling himself "son of man". Spirit filled believers today not only have that same anointing but also the power of the resurrection as is clearly indicated by the Apostle Paul:

> *And if the Spirit of him who raised Jesus from the dead is living in you, he who raised Christ from the dead will also* **give life to your mortal bodies** *through his Spirit, who lives in you.* (Romans 8:11, NIV)

Christ makes it clear, in His last words to His disciples after His resurrection and before He ascended, that he expects his believing followers to accept His Spirit and His anointing and act accordingly. He also said He had much more to teach them and us even though He was leaving earth. Surely He knew that both scientific and Rhema (spoken word of

God) revelation would be among his "future teaching tools". (See John 16:12-15 and Mark 16:16-19.)

His own words indicate that Jesus expects us to intentionally follow His **model** of bringing the sick, broken-hearted and infirm into manifested health. He modeled a process we can employ. I'm quite certain I would not be alive today were there not anointed "believing believers" who were obedient to Christ's admonishment cited above. For those wanting to "lock cancer out of their lives", I believe it critical to understand the power available to us through Christ's resurrection. To stop at the cross belittles the "living Christ" and *"Christ in us the hope of glory"* (Colossians 1:27).

It is critical that we look at Jesus' healing ministry if we are to get past the frustrations of "hoping against hope", "desperate prayer list rituals", and impotent "altar calls" marred by the skepticism of non-believers or, worse, of "unbelieving believers"– who figuratively tear pages out of their Bibles because they build doctrine from circumstances rather than God's Word. We must help each other live in health and wholeness through compassion rather than sympathy. God is not limited by what we see going on in the physical world. Both His Word and His science– indeed his nature– give us this truth. Shortly, we take a more focused look at what Quantum Mechanics will teach us about *"faith being the substance of things hoped for"* (Hebrews 11:1).

How is Healing a Done Deal ?

Again, recall my early morning "download" from God, "The Bible is True". The truth is that we must "discern the body of Jesus" when He took the stripes on His back to understand that **His blood shed on the cross to atone for the sins of the world was not all He accomplished in that great act.** He took the scourging on his body with the cat of nine tails to secure our bodily healing and his soul was *"poured out unto death"* (Isaiah 53:12) on the cross for our soul healing as his precious blood poured forth to redeem us from sin.

Three profound Scriptures verify the truth I just described. Please note the tenses in the following "three witnesses":

Isaiah 53:5

But He was wounded for our transgressions, He was bruised for our guilt and iniquities; the chastisement [needful to obtain] peace and well being for us was upon Him, and with the stripes [that wounded] Him we **are healed and made whole.** (Present tense)

1 Peter 2:24

He personally bore our sins in His [own] body on the tree [as on an altar and offered Himself on it], that we might die (cease to exist) to sin and live to righteousness. By His wounds **you have been healed**. (Past tense)

Matthew 8:17

And thus He fulfilled what was spoken by the prophet Isaiah, He Himself took [in order to carry away] our weaknesses and infirmities and **bore away our diseases.** (Past tense)

The past and present verb tenses used by Holy Spirit in these Scriptures indicates that healing is, in truth, "a done deal". Because many Christians are unaware of their full atonement– that is body, soul and spirit, I'm compelled to share that T.J. McCrossan, the great Greek scholar, who wrote *Bodily Healing and the Atonement,* teaches that the Greek word for "healed" referenced by Peter above and in the *Septuagint* (Greek version of the Old Testament) translation of Isaiah above both use the Greek word, *iaomai,* a verb that **ALWAYS** speaks of **physical healing** in the New Testament. It is used 28 times in the New Testament and always in connection with physical healing.[3]

I could spend pages quoting great Greek and Hebrew scholars on this topic. I won't, but I implore you to study for yourself resources in Appendix One. My purpose is to encourage my believing readers to understand that physical healing is as much of our birthright as forgiveness of our sin when we fully discern the body of Christ– when we understand that celebrating Holy Communion is recognizing the completed work of our Lord.

This understanding is essential, as Rev. Cheryl Schang observes, "It's almost impossible to use your faith if you think you are trying to get God to do something He might not want to do. It's easy to use your faith if you realize that all you must do is use your words to enforce what God has already done . . . You are not operating in presumption. It does not offend God . . . The Bible is clear that God wants you healed – here – in this life-time." [4] Schang's words take me back to Pastor Tom's powerful prayers.

Earlier I suggested you stop and read Psalms 103:1-5. It's pertinent here as well.

> Bless the LORD, O my soul: and all that is within me, bless his holy name.
> Bless the LORD, O my soul, and forget not all his benefits:
> Who forgives **all** thine iniquities; who heals **all** thy diseases;
> Who redeems thy life from destruction; who crowns thee with loving kindness and tender mercies;
> Who satisfies thy mouth with good things; so that thy youth is renewed like the eagle's. (KJV)

Psalms 103 speaks in present tense. Isaiah 53:5 cited earlier speaks in past tense. Both are Old Testament prophesy of Christ's accomplishments for us. There are no time constraints in the Kingdom of God . . . no tense exists. In Christ, healing is "a done deal" . . . mine, yours, ALL. Rebirth in Christ creates heirs to both healing and deliverance.

It is fair to ask, then, why are "Believers in Christ" still dealing with sickness? Are we too often like the heir unaware of the divine "safety deposit box" setting in our name loaded with healing treasure? I am compelled to look at what the Apostle Paul wrote in his first letter to the Corinthians explaining the danger to 'believers" there who were not discerning the body of the Lord. He wrote in 1 Corinthians 11:29-31, ASV:

> For he that eats and drinks, eats and drinks judgment unto himself, **if he discern not the body.**

For this cause many among you are weak and sickly, and not a few sleep.

Read what T.J. McCrossan explains about Paul's admonishment: "Yes, healing is in the Atonement, but no saint (believer) is held guilty in God's sight who fails for any reason to discern this fact; **he only suffers himself**." [5] McCrossan is saying that God is not punishing people with sickness if they don't discern the body, however, if we don't discern our inheritance, we can't benefit from it.

When the "C word" came into my life, I'd been a Christian for nearly 50 years and raised in a church that celebrated Communion every single Sunday; yet, I never discerned the body until I studied those who taught from the original language of the Scripture Canon. I always valued the sacrament and meant to approach it reverently, but I never fully understood the birthright my Lord had paid for. None of us could ever be "worthy" of any of the inheritance Christ passes to us, but it is ours nevertheless IF we realize what we have.

In her insightful book, *Heal Them All,* Rev. Cheryl Schang helps us "discern Christ's body" through an understanding of the "Passover Lamb" which was and is a "metaphor" of Christ. She points out the importance of Scripture using the metaphor in "veiling the mystery so that satan would not be able to figure out that he'd better not allow Jesus to be crucified." Schang goes on to explain that, like a spotless, innocent sacrificial lamb that the Hebrews sacrificed for redemption, Jesus "was morally spotless, but his picture did not match the picture of the Passover lamb in one important way. Jesus was tortured and mutilated before his death more than any other man." (Isaiah 52:14) [6]

Schang explains further, "When the lamb was offered as a sacrifice, it was killed in the most humane way . . . As we know, that does not match the picture of Jesus' experience. He did not die a painless death. Why this deviation? The truth is **Jesus could have died a painless death to give you eternal life.** All that was required was His life in exchange for yours. He could have fulfilled the type and shadow of the sacrifices without suffering. He could have completed the plan for your eternal life without the scourge of the Roman whip . . .. But He didn't. '**He was wounded so that you could be healed'."** [7]

Continuing, Rev. Schang asks, "Do you understand that it was not His suffering that brought you eternal life? It was His death that brought you eternal life. His **suffering** brought you healing, '*By His stripes you are healed*' (Isaiah 53:5). Jesus did not just replace the Old Covenant with a New Covenant; He replaced it with a new and improved version. The New Covenant had healing built into it." [8]

When I learned this Scriptural truth, it literally amounted to "stepping out of a dark shadow".

Because the subject of Holy Communion is seminal to healing and health, please bear with me for one more observation. I want to be sensitive to my readers for whom the concept of bodily healing in the atonement is new. My purpose is to give you information from several sources so you can study further. Certainly many of you may be thinking of earthly circumstances that just don't seem to mesh with the concept of discerning the body of Christ even though you long ago discerned the atoning blood of Jesus for remission of the sins of all who accept Him as Lord. On the other hand, some readers may have no experience with the concepts I am discussing here. I implore you to look at this Lamb, this Christ, and seek a greater discernment of the atoning sacrifice.

The more we learn about quantum mechanics and the power of our own intent matching God's intent, the more we must open up to the mysteries of Scripture– indeed the promises of God's own Word and the innate power of our own gratitude (*Eucharisteo*) that must be rooted in full discernment of our blessings. It's time to open that treasure box we already have.

Pastor Joseph Prince, in his book, *Health and Wholeness Through Holy Communion,* also examines Paul's admonishment to the Church at Corinth (cited above) pointing out that Paul said in verse 30, "for this cause" or "for this reason" depending on translation but always singular (not causes). "Paul had singled out this **one reason** as the cause of sickness and, ultimately, premature death for many Christians. [9] "And what was this reason?" asked Prince. "It was not discerning the Lord's body". Prince concludes, "It means that they did not know why they were partaking of the body when they came to the table. They had no idea why they were eating the bread. And this was the reason they were not receiving the divine life of their Savior, causing them to be weak and sick, and to die prematurely."[10]

The Appendix Two of this book includes more resources to help you understand the power of Holy Communion. It is truly the "meal that heals". I celebrate it daily at home. I believe you will find that Holy Eucharist or Holy Communion explains perfectly the power of gratitude in healing and wholeness. Jesus modeled a grateful spirit constantly in his earthly ministry such as before raising Lazarus (John 11:41) and before feeding thousands from a few loaves and fishes. (John 6:5-14) Later, I will discuss an amazing scientific demonstration of the influence of "gratitude" upon water molecules remembering that our bodies are 70+% water.

It is powerful to be constantly thanking God for the manifestation of our healing even before we "see" it. We are changed in body, soul and spirit through honestly grateful expression because science and Scripture merge within the power of gratitude. A careful reading of the New Testament reveals many revelations regarding Holy Communion. Watch for the miracles that occur after the "breaking of bread" like, for example, the opening of the two disciples' eyes on the Road to Emmaeus (see Luke 24:30-31) and Paul's and others survival of a devastating shipwreck (Acts 27:34-38).

Inter-active Miracles Manifest Wholeness

Let's examine Biblical healing of both body and soul. The first Scripture I want to point out is not a miracle at the hands of Jesus, but one enacted by Jesus's "inner circle" disciples, Peter and John, whom no one could argue were in any way "divine". They were obviously praying men full of faith and anointed by Holy Spirit which are all qualities available to us as we see in Acts 3:1-9:

> *And Peter and John were going up at the same time to the temple, at the hour of the prayer, the ninth hour,*
> *and a certain man, being lame from the womb of his mother, was being carried, whom they were laying every day at the gate of the temple, called Beautiful, to ask a* **kindness** *from those entering into the temple*
> *who, having seen Peter and John about to go into the temple, was begging to receive a* **kindness**.
> *And Peter, having looked steadfastly toward him with John, said, 'Look toward us;' and he was giving heed to them, looking to receive something from them;*
> *and Peter said, 'Silver and gold I have none, but what I have, that I give to thee; in the name of Jesus Christ of Nazareth, rise up and be walking.'*
> *And having seized him by the right hand, he raised him up, and presently his feet and ankles were strengthened, 8 and springing up, he stood, and was walking, and did enter with them into the temple, walking and springing, and praising God; 9 and all the people saw him walking and praising God.* (YLT)

How did these two men lead this lame man to health? Did the lame man do anything? Yes, the lame man **expected** or **intended** to receive something from the disciples. The disciples freely **gave what they had** which was the anointing "in the name of Jesus of Nazareth". Did the disciples beg God to heal the man? NO! Apparently, they "properly discerned the body of the Lord" and knew healing had already been accomplished. They touched the man, seizing his hand, and confidently commanded him to *"rise up and be walking"*. He participated in the miracle. They, too, **expected** or **intended** for something to happen as this command implies– they **intended for the man's healing to manifest.** They **commanded a specific action and moved in it**. Their actions modeled effective prayer for healing that applies now as then. They offered compassion with intent to bring forth healing.

Then, the man went *"springing, walking, and praising God"* indicating that this man was healed in more than his body but also in his soul. He was filled with joy having received wholeness allowing him not only to walk but also to express that joy by *"springing"* and he showed his spiritual health by *"praising God"*. Please realize that this man was a Jew and, having been lame *"from the womb of his mother"*, meant that he had been considered cursed (see Deuteronomy 28 entire chapter). As a result he surely had been wounded in soul throughout life - maligned because Hebrew culture made little distinction between sin and sickness.

Looking at another "miracle", we will consider the question of why some people who are prayed for are not healed or why some have physical healing manifest but only temporarily. HOW Jesus led people to their health answers these questions. The Roman centurion's servant even amazed Jesus. Matthew 8:5-10 and 13 tells the story:

> And Jesus having entered into Capernaum, there came to him a centurion calling upon him, and saying, 'Sir, my young man hath been laid in the house a paralytic, fearfully afflicted,' and Jesus said to him, 'I, having come, will heal him.' And the centurion answering said, 'Sir, I am not worthy that thou may enter under my roof, **but only say a word**, and my servant shall be healed; for I also am a man under authority, having under myself soldiers, and I say to this one, Go, and he goes, and to another, Be coming, and he comes, and to my servant, Do this, and he does it.' And Jesus having heard, did wonder, and said to those following, 'Verily I say to you, not even in Israel so great faith have I found. (YLT)
>
> And Jesus said to the centurion, 'Go, and as thou didst believe let it be to thee;' and his young man was healed in **that hour**.

What hour? The hour the healing words were spoken in a place remote from the person who was healed. Apparently prayer with bold intention can have impact remotely and instantly. Jesus ministered as an anointed human being with authority according to the laws (principles) of the universe that never change? Remember that He knew the laws because we know He knew God's Word - both logos (written Scriptures) and Rhema (God's voice).

What did Jesus *"wonder"* about in verse ten above? Jesus basically marveled at the centurion's grasp of reality beyond that which could be seen and confirmed. Jesus marveled that the centurion understood that authority and spoken words actually accomplish things - even remotely located things. The Centurion was sensing the reality we are now discovering through quantum physics– specifically the power of focus and intent.

WOW! Could Jesus not have spoken a word that healed every sick person in all of Israel? Couldn't He have just lined up people and spoken a word and had all of them physically healed instantly? Talk about an expedient "prayer line". Apparently He could have because He did it in the case just cited and we know he was/is *"no respecter of persons"* (Acts 10:34). However, God did not instruct Him to heal everyone with a quick word. In His ministry, Jesus **treated each one as a unique person.** How he ministered teaches us about wholeness. Healing isn't "enough" for our loving Father God. He wants us to be "in health".

In other cases, like the woman with the issue of blood, Jesus is again amazed at the faith of one healed. Mark 5:25-34 relates the story:

> *And there was a woman who had had a flow of blood for twelve years,*
> *And who had endured much suffering under [the hands of] many physicians and had spent all that she had, and was no better but instead grew worse.*
> *She had heard the reports concerning Jesus, and she came up behind Him in the throng and touched His garment,*
> *For she kept saying, If I only touch His garments, I shall be restored to health.*

And immediately her flow of blood was dried up at the source, and [suddenly] she felt in her body that she was healed of her [distressing] ailment.

And Jesus, recognizing in Himself that the power proceeding from Him had gone forth, turned around immediately in the crowd and said, Who touched My clothes?

And the disciples kept saying to Him, You see the crowd pressing hard around You from all sides, and You ask, Who touched Me?

Still He kept looking around to see her who had done it.

But the woman, knowing what had been done for her, though alarmed and frightened and trembling, fell down before Him and told Him the whole truth.

And He said to her, Daughter, your faith (your trust and confidence in Me, springing from faith in God) has restored you to health. Go in (into) peace and be continually healed and freed from your [distressing bodily] disease.

Was this woman's soul healed along with her body even though Jesus was unaware of the healing until He *"realized that power had gone out of Him"*? Certainly! Again, context is important. This Jewish woman had dealt with a bleeding issue twelve years. Holy Spirit focuses on the time span as well as her disappointment in human doctors pointing out she had even grown worse. She was also damaged financially. Considered "unclean" by her culture, she took a huge risk coming out in public. Soul wounds galore! Yet, she was healed "at the source". I suggest that, because she had grown worse with physical treatment rather than better, "the source" of her ailment was her soul wounds. Jesus seems to confirm this conclusion when he stresses she should "go in **peace**" and be "**continually healed**" and freed from a "**distressing** bodily disease".

Gratitude Powers Determination

Could this woman's story teach us that intent to be healed impacts our healing both in body and soul? It is obvious that this woman was intent.

She was willing to risk being publicly maligned in order to partake of the power of Jesus's anointing. This story is often referenced in sermons to teach "having (even conjuring up) enough faith to be healed"; however, could not the main lesson in this story really be about faithful persistence and earnest intent?

Dr. Bernie Siegel writes, "The resolve to do whatever is necessary, including opening up the unconscious, is one of the first requirements for being an exceptional patient." [11] Siegel's subject is essentially the qualities he has observed in patients over the years who overcame life threatening illness. Dr. Siegel's "exceptional patients", much like the woman with the issue of blood, are the ones willing to risk even shame if it brings them back to health. These are the patients whose health is restored.

Marilyn Hickey, an evangelist now in her eighties and long ago healed of cancer herself, still energetically ministers worldwide. In her very encouraging teaching CD, "Eight Ways God Heals", Marilyn stresses that it is the "violent people who get their healing". "Violent people" would be those as persistent as the woman with the issue of blood who was healed by risking, focusing, decreeing, intending and touching the hem of Jesus' garment. [12]

Katie Souza, whose revelation regarding soul healing provides an expedient process I share later, points out that this Jewish woman obviously knew Scripture well. *A specific* part of God's Word likely empowered this woman's faithful persistence. It is Malachi 4:2 which says: *But unto you who revere and worshipfully fear My name shall the Sun of Righteousness arise with **healing in His wings** and His beams, and you shall go forth and gambol like calves [released] from the stall and leap for joy.*

Souza explains that "wings" in this Scripture refer to the tassels on the corners of the prayer shawl Jewish teachers wore in Jesus' day. The woman knew in her soul that there was healing in those "wings" because she believed Jesus was the "sent one" referred to as the "Sun of Righteousness". The "power" that went from Jesus to the woman is the Greek word, dunamis, which is "glory light" or the "beams" in the Malachi Scripture. It is also the power within Jesus' resurrection. [13]

This woman had a specific Scripture to cling too just like I had the one the fencing contractor shared with me (James 5:14). The Word of God is ALWAYS powerful. If you are seeking healing, I implore you to stand on specific Scriptures. You can find these "Healing Scriptures" on my blog, www.slamthedooroncancer.com, in Appendix One and in audio on my blog, www.realhealthhope.com.

Jesus Originated Inter-Active Miracles

In Luke 5:12-14 we walk with Jesus:

> *While Jesus was in one of the towns, a man came along who was covered with leprosy. When he saw Jesus, he fell with his face to the ground and begged him, "Lord, if you are willing, you can make me clean."*
>
> ***Jesus reached out his hand and touched the man. "I am willing," he said. "Be clean!" And immediately the leprosy left him.***
>
> *Then Jesus ordered him, "Don't tell anyone, but go, show yourself to the priest and offer the sacrifices that Moses commanded for your cleansing, as a **testimony to them**." (NIV)*

Lepers were ostracized through fear of contagion. This man had probably not felt the touch of another human being for a very long time. Touch is important to our soul (emotional) health. This leper was unsure if Jesus would give him the time of day because he said, "**If** you are willing", but he was **sure** in faith that Jesus **could** heal him. Jesus could have just spoken a word as demonstrated with the Centurion's servant; yet He touched the man without hesitation healing his soul, which facilitated a healed body. The man was clean inside and out. Jesus commanded it knowing the source of disease and using His spiritual authority. Then, to make sure this man's spiritual life was sound, Jesus sent him to **do** something that would fulfill spiritual law - something "normal" in his culture. This man hadn't done anything "normal" for a long time. His was an inter-active miracle.

Jesus models a "healing ministry" of compassion - never "detached" or "routine". The "process" in every case met the needs of the person before Him.

In Luke 17:11-19 we read the story of the ten lepers. Only one of these men, not even a Jew, returns to thank Jesus and praise God. Of these ten men, which do you think will remain in health? Which was made whole? We have already mentioned the power of gratitude and will visit it again.

In Mark 2:1-12, we read about four friends who lower a paralytic through a roof into the midst of the crowd around Jesus. Jesus offended the "religious" leaders present saying to the man, "Your sins are forgiven" instead of "your body is healed". Jesus answers the leaders basically saying, "what's the difference?" which, I believe, clarifies that a wounded soul and infirm body are one problem as my own story illustrates.

In John 5:5-15, we read about a crippled man in a crowd who for 38 years had gathered with others at the Pool of Bethesda focused on an occasional seemingly random chance at healing. Jesus obviously walked this route to the temple often but the man had never asked Him for healing. (We know because Jesus never turned anyone down.) When Jesus asks him if he wants to get well, the man only expresses self-pity at having no man to help him beat others to the healing pool. Jesus interrupts his whining saying, *"take up your bed and go"*, but sees him later and says, *"See, you are well and strong; do no more sin for fear a worse thing comes to you"*. Whining and self-pity are sinful and unproductive.

Theologian Harold Eberle teaches, "Self pity is a negative force . . . Self pity is the positioning of one's heart in a selfish manner, which draws – or steals – the energy of other people. It is a form of lust or coveting of other people's strength and love." [14] Obviously the man at the pool coveted other people's helpers.

Could this story be in the canon to teach the link between sickness and insidious sin such as self-pity? I am not implying that every sick person embodies self-pity but that it can sneak into our souls as the enemy sends debilitating thoughts we fail to take captive.

People pray a lot of "hope against hope" prayer without understanding the individual situation they are praying into and, if they don't see the person return to health, they often make up some excuse for God. **We too often overlook that a great many diseased bodies have dis-eased souls living within them.** We MUST deal with the wounded soul before a healed body can sustain recovery as Jesus's ministry modeled. I am not accusing the sick of sin. I am accusing the enemy of accusing, stealing, lying, and convincing. I've experienced it and I know it's real and many who successfully minister to the sick know the spiritual roots of disease must be dealt with every single time.

Notes:

Section II

Harnessing Your Emotional Power for Healing

"Emotions are real—they exist in time and space and are located through-out our minds and bodies . . . Emotions are at the nexus between matter and mind, going back and forth between the two and influencing both."
Dr. Candace Pert, PhD, biochemist, in *Molecules of Emotion*.

five

Cool Mind, Cool Body

Throughout his book, *A More Excellent Way to Be in Health,* Dr. Henry W. Wright discusses countless cases linking specific emotional roots with certain diseases. Most people have some idea that worry, stress, and anxiety can cause disease, but few understand that wounds from unforgiven sin **against us** can prohibit wholeness of body, soul and spirit.[1] Sometimes people receive manifestation of their physical healing but lose it because their soul remains wounded. "Remission failure" comes to my mind regarding such recurrence. Let us examine blocks to healing from a scientific perspective.

Dr. Johanna Budwig, brilliant scientist and practitioner throughout the 1900's, was very successful in treating cancer through the science of her "oil/protein protocol" which we will examine closely later. She recognized that "we cannot reduce the cancer entirely to the cells". In her book, *Cancer– The Problem and The Solution,* she said, "It is very important to view the person as a unit consisting of body, soul, and psyche." [2] [She referred to spirit as "soul" and soul as "psyche".]

Dr. Budwig continued, "When a healing seemed stalled, I would ask whether the patient is Catholic or Lutheran." (The two choices in her native Germany.) And often the patients proceed to tell me for instance how much they are **troubled** by the fact that they have not been to confession for some time. Then I tell the patients that before they return in four weeks, they should go to confession and speak openly with their priest." **She obviously realized that a soul in which guilt or other sin was unresolved would block physical healing.** Regarding children, Budwig observed that stress around them, sin against them, and doctors not giving credence to their reports of trauma or physical injury often emotionally blocked their physical healing.[3]

We've noted that there remains a tension in "medical science" surrounding the mind-body interface. Jesus recognized this interface as we have seen through examining several miracles. He also told his disciples before leaving them: *I have much more to say to you, more than you can now bear. But when the Spirit comes He will guide you into all truth.* (John 16:13, NIV)

Surely he knew that the science we discuss today would be revealed eventually. Some of that very science, it would seem, is that revealed through the work of Dr. Candace Pert, PhD, who, like Dr Budwig, is also a brilliant and courageous biochemist and researcher under appreciated by the "conventional medical system".

Since 1970, when Pert discovered the "opiate receptors" on cell membranes, medical science has been forced, reluctantly, to look up from Cartesian (from DesCartes) dogma. Can the discovery of tiny receptors on cell membranes have such an impact? Yes, because, as Dr. Pert explains, "I found a way to measure it and thereby prove its existence. ["It" being the mind-body interface.] Measurement! It is the very foundation of modern scientific method, the means by which the material world is admitted into existence. Unless we can measure something, science won't concede it exists, which is why science refuses to deal with such 'non-things' as the emotions, the mind, the soul, or the spirit." [4]

The opiate receptors fit both narcotic (such as morphine) and endogenous (such as endorphin) molecules that alter mood, pain etc. These receptors receive the biochemically transported "molecules of emotion" to every body cell and the cells respond in specific physical ways. **It is an absolutely proven dynamic two-way communication between body and soul.**

There are thousands of receptors on our cell membranes specifically designed to fit particular biochemical molecules, like a lock receiving a key. Examples are insulin, hormones, neuropeptides, etc. The significance of the opiate receptor is that **the cell membrane holds a receptor for molecules stimulated by specific emotions.** In Dr. Pert's own words, "the neuropeptides and their receptors are the **substrates of the emotions and they are in constant communication with the immune system**, the mechanism through which health and disease are created." She continues, "Think of (stress related disease) in terms of an information overload, a situation in which the mind-body network is so taxed by unprocessed sensory input in the form of **suppressed trauma or undigested emotions** that it has become bogged down and cannot flow freely, sometimes even working against itself, at cross-purposes." [5]

As a scientist, Dr. Pert speaks to the same soul healing lessons we find in the scriptural healing accounts when we see Jesus not settling for a quick fix bodily healing but also making sure of soul healing as well. His goal was and is obviously wholeness. Dr. Pert concludes, "Aim for emotional wholeness. When you're upset or feeling sick, try to get to the bottom of your feelings. Figure out what's really eating you. **Always tell the truth to yourself.**" [6]

Here is a "graphic analogy" from Dr. Pert: "Visualize the following: If the cell is the engine that drives all life, then the receptors are the buttons on the control panel of that engine, and the ligand (attached atom or molecule) is the finger that pushes that button and things get started." [7]

Dr. Pert is saying "molecules of emotion" push our buttons at the cellular level where tumors happen and our immune system is drawn into the fray. Think of the body's familiar responses to emotions such as anger, embarrassment, fear and other "INSULTS". We all know the "feelings" resulting and we also know the physical manifestations that can include (but not be limited to) our faces getting either hot red or ashen white depending on the emotional stimulus.

These things happen because of chemicals spilled into our blood stream that fit receptors on our cell membranes and impact every single cell function on every single body cell. Most of these chemicals are part of our "first response protection system"—our immune system. Inflammation is part of this process and it is meant to be temporarily helpful—fight or flight. Inflammation is part of the wound fighting process-either internally or externally but never permanently.

The danger to our body cells comes from sustained dumping of these strong chemicals into our blood and then into our cells. The inflammation becomes a "wild fire" and cells respond abnormally so that we experience internal "wounds that won't heal" because fuel continues to be poured on the fire. [8]

These fires can manifest in various body tissues (groups of cells) but the basic cause must be addressed regardless of the site of that wound which can become a malignancy. Again, recall that the word "malign" is the root word for malignancy. Response to being chronically maligned can become malignancy at the cellular level. "Soul wounds" can be suppressed painful memories that recycle the biochemical fuel feeding disease. Learning to process "insult" and "offense" in a healthy way, indeed with love, is critical for avoiding dis-ease as we saw in our discussion of the "pure laws of health". Everything Jesus teaches us applies to this "anti-offense love" as does mind-body scientific reality.

Soul Wounds are the Enemy's Campsite

In Dr. Pert's second book, *Everything You Need to Know to Feel Go(o)d*, she offers fresh insight, "Whether your memories are conscious or not is mediated by the molecules of emotion. They decide what becomes a thought rising to the surface and what remains buried deeply in your body. What this means is that much of memory is emotion driven, not conscious, although it can sometimes be *made* conscious by **intention**. The emotions that you're able to experience can bring a recollection to the surface; if your feelings are suppressed, however, they can bury that same memory far below your awareness where it can affect your perceptions, decisions, behavior, and even **health**, all unconsciously. Buried, painful emotions from the past make up what some psychologists and healers call a person's 'core emotional trauma'." [9]

Jesus was certainly aware of every person's "core emotional trauma" which I've been referring to as "soul wounds". He was always listening for a Rhema word from Father God. Soul wounds can be the result of trauma such as a serious accident, abuse, neglect, etc. They can also be the result of sin– our own or sin against us. Please don't react to the word "sin" as though it is too legalistic, judgmental, or religious. Sin is a word to define the intentional or unintentional "breaking of pure laws" such as love, work, and stewardship we discussed earlier. Trauma and sin are the principle causes of "soul wounds" or "core emotional trauma". I am not encouraging you to become "guilt ridden" or "sin conscious" because that leads to "religious legalism" which is very destructive. I am simply attempting to examine the actual physical impact of emotional separation from our Creator's "pure laws"—I do not mean "pure rules" but rather "principles by which relationship with our Creator are maintained thereby allowing us to experience wholeness". We are wired for relationship with God so that issues in life short-circuiting that connection must be dealt with. God is not mad at us. He just needs us to give Him our "junk in our trunk".

Earlier, I transparently shared my own "soul wounds" that twice underpinned the cancerous assault on my pancreas. I also shared the James Chapter Five prayer and oil service that set me on the road to soul healing as a pre-requisite for bodily healing even before I had a clue about the mind-body connection. Thank God because, medically speaking, I didn't have enough pancreas left to survive a second relapse. My healing had to become wholeness so it would last. My case is not unusual. Relapse is almost expected in treating cancer which appears to be why the medical term is never "cure" but "remission"– except when "donate to find a cure" is part of the conversation. I've already shared my basis for questioning the term "remission". Words are important, as I will soon examine in more depth.

As I shared before, God gave me a "connect the dots" miracle requiring my interaction or "co-laboring" with Him. Remember that Jesus often gave instructions to those He ministered to for healing like "go wash in the pool of Siloam" or "go show yourself to the priests". One morning well past my second bout of pancreatic surgery, I was doing something very unusual for me - holding a TV remote and channel surfing with no particular goal. I watch very little TV except, during my post-op recovery, I was much encouraged by both the Joyce Meyer and Marilyn Hickey Shows. By this time I was fairly active; yet, there I was on the sofa compelled to search for something with no idea what.

Suddenly, the words, "It's Supernatural" flashed across the "guide grid" and I curiously hit the button. Sid Roth, the host, was interviewing an attractive young woman and her story was riveting. Looking like an angel, she transparently discussed her many years "on the street" dealing and doing drugs, cooking dope, holding guns to people's heads collecting drug money, fighting with outlaw bikers, being repeatedly thrown into federal prison lockdown for fighting. Then Sid asked her about her ministry and I was floored because I hadn't yet gotten past her past. I thought, "If she has a viable ministry, it has to be God!"

This young woman was Katie Souza and her now internationally respected ministry is Expected End Ministries named after Jeremiah 29:11: *For I know the thoughts that I think toward you, says the Lord, thoughts of peace, and not of evil, **to give you an Expected End.*** (KJV)

She also mentioned her book based on that Scripture entitled, *The Captivity Series,* mainly targeted at helping prisoners, whom she lovingly calls "her peeps", rebuild their lives. Sid mentioned the book then asked her about her teaching series called "The Healing School". By then I was quite curious. Obviously, the study of healing had been my life and death focus for some time and I remained perplexed by the question of why some who were prayed for did not have healing manifest. Katie was talking about "soul wounds" blocking physical healing. This is a concept I had never put into words even though I knew the root of my own illness had been a wounded soul ever since my "pancreas vision" the night after my oil service.

A visitor to Katie Souza's ministry website at www.expectedendministries.com, can actually listen to audio or watch video of some pretty amazing teaching. I particularly encourage you to watch her free teaching on "Blocked Healing" by clicking "Media" and then "Teaching". You may then want to go to some of her foundational teaching such as "Kingdom of the Son" which includes a great deal of Scriptural basis for particular soul wounds causing the physical inflammation I touched on earlier.

What is the revelation upon which this most unlikely ministry is built? It's JESUS– the blood, the resurrection and something most Christians know little about– the dunamis power of the resurrection. I will introduce the basics, and encourage you to pursue it further. Of course Souza's own story illustrates the power of her revelation. Who would doubt that her former life was a soul-wounding journey, yet she has been miraculously healed of several physical diseases (including lupus) as a result of her revelation. God teaches us the power of testimony and Expected End Ministries is rich in faith building testimony.

The basic precept of Souza's teaching is that trauma or sin inflicts wounds on our souls embedding memories much as Dr. Pert scientifically describes. Our bodies hold those damaging and inflammatory memories because every trauma or sin wounds our soul. We hold onto unforgiveness, bitterness, resentment, hatred, offense, envy, fear, or other damaging emotional memories. Also, we can have images of idols, as Souza says, "Burned onto our souls" or into our memories from obsessions with things we have let become too important in our lives. Sometimes we repeatedly recycle hurtful memories through our consciousness. Sometimes we push them down and refuse to deal with them. I did both. Sometimes we become addicts. I became a workaholic, I believe, to maintain distraction from dealing with my soul wounds.

In every case, however, our bodies continue to biochemically respond to the stress. But here's the next revelation. Soul wounds give the enemy of our souls a legal place to camp out which keeps the sin, trauma, and "offense" churning within us. Sin is his domain. We can't kick him out if we "keep his campfire burning". He can "burn us up" physically using emotional fuel. Does the word "inflammation" come to mind? Souza makes the connection in her teaching on "Staying Unoffendable".

What must we do to get our souls healed? Jesus told us: *But I say to you who are hearing, Love your enemies, do good to those hating you.* (Luke 6:27, YLT)

Katie Souza teaches us to repent for (reverse direction from) the sin that has caused our soul wounds as we follow the admonition of the Lord's words. This is essentially impossible without consciously applying the atoning love of His blood on the sin that caused our wounds. It is critical that we also repent and intently apply the blood of Jesus on those who have sinned against us. Our focus on repenting and forgiving is honest love– the basis for honest forgiving. Jesus makes the need to forgive quite plain in Mark 11:25: *And whenever you stand praying, if you have anything against anyone, forgive him and let it drop (leave it, let it go), in order that your Father Who is in heaven may also forgive you your [own] failings and shortcomings and let them drop.*

Also remember that power and energy follow our focus just like it did for the woman with the issue of blood. Quantum physics is showing us the power of our intent and Scripture shows us that intent must be from our hearts and not just verbal. We may never forget what we've forgiven; however focusing on our healing instead of the "dis-ease" is ALWAYS where the power is. Actually, focusing on Jesus, the Healer, rather than the sought after healing is where the healing power arises as it did for the woman with the issue of blood. I found it amazing how memories of past hurts faded away once I reversed my focus through repenting.

When we aren't sure what we might need to repent for, we must ask God to tell us and listen quietly to receive the needed insight. After we have forgiven and repented for the specific sins and offenses that have wounded our souls, we wait for a feeling of peace or a release. Then, we begin to focus on the dunamis power or glory light of Jesus' resurrection. We focus this incomparable power and light on our soul wounds (painful memories) every time they arise because light heals in both the natural and the spiritual realm.

Once our soul wounds are healed, we **verbally** kick the enemy out of our souls and, thereby, out of our bodies because he no longer has a legal right to be there. Just firmly command him to leave and not return **in the mighty name of Jesus**. Don't give this defeated enemy much attention just evict him. Once he knows you are aware of who you are in Christ, this enemy knows he's toast. Remember, the Apostle Paul said, *"I want to know Him and the power of His resurrection"* (Phil 3:10). That power is dunamis and it gives us "excellence of soul".

The enemy is not omniscient, omnipresent or equal to God in any way. There are quasi "Christian" organizations that have, for generations, published their own "Bibles" teaching an equally powerful tension between God and satan. In fact, if your heritage includes "brotherhood" or "sisterhood" in such an organization (as mine did), you may have generational soul wounds from that association. Ask God if you have generational issues to repent for even if you were never involved directly yourself or your ancestor was unaware of the occult (satan glorification) roots of such involvement. Remember, the enemy is a tricky counterfeiter. We discussed earlier that we are not slaves to our DNA, which includes the damage done by any occult involvement of our ancestors. Generational curses are not "our burden to bear" in our DNA if we **purposely intend** otherwise.

Notes:

six

Using The Power of Intention

The scientist, Masaru Emoto, in his book entitled *Hidden Messages in Water,* experimented with focused prayer as well as the impact of isolated words on water. Emoto cites an experiment in which a large group of "prayer warriors" went to the largest lake in Japan, which was grossly polluted at the time. They surrounded the lake praying with **focused intent** for its purification, which was achieved. Water samples verified lake conditions before and after prayer. [1] This "experiment" is Quantum Mechanics at work and I believe we see it at work in Jesus' ministry which can help us understand Scriptures like Ephesians 3:20: *Now to Him Who,* **by (in consequence of) the [action of His] power that is at work within us**, *is able to [carry out His purpose and] do superabundantly, far over and above all that we [dare] ask or think [infinitely beyond our highest prayers, desires, thoughts, hopes, or dreams].*

Remember the healing miracle (Matthew 8:5-13) in which a Roman Centurion amazed Jesus by asking Him *"to say the word only"* and his servant would be healed. He was correct. Jesus did just that and the servant was healed at *"that very same hour"* although Jesus was not in the same physical "space" as the ill servant. Jesus *"wondered"* at the soldier's *"faith"*; however, I believe that Jesus was also amazed that the Centurion had a practical inkling of quantum mechanics. Jesus remarked to the crowd about the Centurion's *"great faith"* and said to the Centurion, *"Go! It will be done just as you believed it would."* "Believing believers", today, call what Jesus did for the Centurion "intercession" which also means, "prayerful intervening".

Looking deeper into this example of the "power of intercessory prayer", there is a profound lesson. There was no fear in the Centurion and, certainly, none in Jesus. There was love for his bondservant in the Centurion and, as Luke describes, Jewish elders reported to Jesus that this Roman officer also *"loves our nation and built our synagogue"*. I contend that the absence of fear (negative energy) and the presence of love (absolutely positive energy) interfaces the physics of heaven and earth within this story. The Centurion, the Jewish elders, and, of course, Jesus absolutely fully intended for that servant to be made whole.

The writer of Hebrews tells us that Jesus is now and ever our intercessor at the right hand of God eternally. Hebrews 7:25 assures us: *Therefore He is able also to save to the uttermost (completely, perfectly, finally, and for all time and eternity) those who come to God through Him, since **He is always living to make petition to God and intercede with Him and intervene for them**.*

Therefore, all reborn in Christ have no basis for fear because we are so loved that God sent His only son to put on flesh, reverse the curse, and "finish" restoration. He arose and went to His heavenly throne and God sent Holy Spirit to counsel, enable, advise, and guide because, again, He **intends** for us to live in *"love, joy, peace, patience, kindness, goodness, faithfulness, gentleness and self-control"* (Galatians 5:22). This is GOOD NEWS indeed! Praying "in the name of Jesus" calls on our divine intercessor.

Intent is Power

Why is this intent a big deal? Why is the presence of love and absence of fear a big deal? Because we are really talking about energy and Dr. Bruce Lipton says it well, "You can live a life of fear or live a life of love. You have the choice! But I can tell you that if you choose to see a world full of love, your body will respond by growing in health." [2] A most important extension of this point is that "to fully thrive, we must not only eliminate the negative stressors, but also actively seek joyful, loving, fulfilling lives that stimulate growth processes." [3] In short, we are not simply "avoiding fear" but we are actively focusing our loving intent on the "miracle" we need. Love rather than fear emits an authoritative energy just like in the Centurion's story.

Paul told the Ephesians:

*In Whom, because of our **faith** in Him, we dare to have the boldness (courage and confidence) of free access (an unreserved approach to God with freedom and without **fear**) well as within ourselves.* (Ephesians 3:12)

The writer of Hebrews said:

*But the just shall live by **faith** [My righteous servant shall live by his conviction respecting man's relationship to God and divine things, and **holy fervor** born of **faith** and conjoined with it]; and if he draws back and shrinks in **fear**, My soul has no delight or pleasure in him.* (Hebrews 10:38)

Energy goes where we pay attention. Intention, I believe, is like a wider bandwidth of attention. And, as we've seen, either fear or faith (pure love) is the wellspring of attention. The Centurion who came to Jesus asking him to *"speak the word only and my servant will be healed"* realized that Jesus authoritatively intended for that healing to happen. He had full faith. He was moving "in love". Fear is like an evil spirit we must choose to admit or deny into the events of our lives. The Centurion did not allow that spirit entry. A great deal of healing energy went to that servant through loving, focused, faithful INTENT. We can do the same thing regarding our own healing and intercession for others. I can tell you, I've experienced the power and joy of such intercession and it is indescribably wonderful.

Everything is Connected and Anything is Possible

David Van Koevering, a physicist and Christian teacher with a powerful personal healing testimony, says, "quantum mechanics appears to describe a universal order that includes us in a very special way. In fact, our minds may enter into nature in a way we had not imagined possible." [4] He discusses the work of several quantum scientists including Einstein and concludes that "Science can demonstrate that atomic and subatomic structures are hooked up and do communicate faster than light. The spiritual realm is about the so-called speed of light and we all are one in that connected cosmic consciousness!". Van Koevering makes a very good argument that "This physical reality is frequency up to the speed of light and the spiritual realm goes all the way up in frequencies all the way to God's full glory. Therefore the spiritual realm is phenomena beyond the speed of light." [5]

What do Van Koevering's observations about the speed of light have to do with prayer and intercession? He is saying that sub-atomic particles moving faster than the speed of light carry our **intent**. We are connected with all of creation at a quantum level and, by our **focus and intent**, we communicate "spiritually". That communication is the same as it was with Jesus, the Centurion, and the servant – powerful! It is powerful for prayer and intercession. It is powerful for bringing God's "kingdom to come on earth as in heaven"– God's "will to be done on earth as in heaven". It is powerful for slamming the door on disease forever! Hosea 4:6 states, *"My people perish for lack of knowledge"*. Quantum Physics is knowledge. Jesus actually demonstrated this truth to us long before we began to glimpse the science of it. I am not talking about magic. I am talking about the power of love. We cannot let the enemy co-opt our power. We have a Kingdom to build "on earth as in Heaven."

Annette Capps, in her booklet, *Quantum Faith,* adds insight to Van Koevering's remarks saying, "In the quantum, subatomic arena, there are only possibilities and probabilities. Things don't work like you think they should. Nothing is there until you look. All that exists is only an infinite number of possibilities. [Remember Jesus said, *"**All things are possible to him that believes."*** (Mark 9:23)] Whereas gravity works whether anyone is present or not (a tree falls down, not up, even if no one observes it), the sub atomic particles traveling faster than light that David Van Koevering discussed are not there unless someone (an observer) looks for them. We can't really know what they are doing, or even if they exist when we are not looking. It is possible that they "are not". 1 Corinthians 1:28 says that

God has chosen the *"things that are not to bring to nought things that are."* [6]

I realize the above paragraph is "brain straining" because it goes against "common sense". Just know that some "old friend" laws (principles), like gravity, work consistently. On the other hand, we now know that all matter is made of vibrating sub-atomic particles moving faster than light (186,000 miles per second) and all matter is inter-connected so that **observing a material object with a certain intent actually changes the physical properties of that object**. This was discovered in light beam experiments in which the light changes back and forth from being particles to being waves depending upon whether the scientist was observing the experiment or not. Surely this science helps us see why sympathy can be damaging? How we look at something changes it including our own bodies and particularly focusing on a part needing restoration.

The writer of Hebrews had a lot to say about this subject that, I believe, Quantum Physics is opening up to us. I quoted the King James translation of Hebrews 11:1 earlier, but I quote the Amplified translation here because it further defines the original Greek:

> *Hebrews 11:1*
> *NOW FAITH is the assurance (the confirmation, the title deed) of the things [we] hope for, being the proof of **things [we] do not see and the conviction of their reality [faith perceiving as real fact what is not revealed to the senses]**.*

> *Hebrews 11:3*
> *By faith we understand that the worlds [during the successive ages] were framed (fashioned, put in order, and equipped for their intended purpose) by the word of God, so that **what we see was not made out of things which are visible**.*

Obviously, I am attempting to provide useful glimpses of the merging of Scripture and Quantum Science knowing the scope of this convergence is limitless. My vision is that my reader will realize that our circumstances are neither determined by a diagnosis, our DNA, nor our dependency on other people including experts - in other words, "facts". Instead, circumstances are determined by "truth" which means we have what we need to set circumstances right. It is not a matter of pumping up our faith, but it is a matter of asking God for our promised *"measure of faith"* (Romans 12:3) and realizing that what our very own Creator tells us in His Word works. In the following Scripture, Jesus had just demonstrated killing a fig tree using words. This Scripture stresses the importance of what we **say,** and then connects the faith carried in words to the necessity of forgiving. Mark 11:21-26 is an empowering Scripture:

> *And Peter having remembered says to him, 'Rabbi, lo, the fig-tree that thou didst curse is dried up.'*
>
> **And Jesus answering says to them, 'Have faith of God; [Note: Note faith "of" rather than ""in" as sometimes wrongly translated.]**
>
> *for verily I say to you, that whoever may say to this mount, Be taken up, and be cast into the sea, and may not doubt in his heart, but may believe that the things that he says do come to pass, it shall be to him whatever he may say.*
>
> *Because of this I say to you, all whatever– praying– ye do ask, believe that ye receive, and it shall be to you.*
>
> *'And whenever ye may stand praying, forgive, if ye have anything against any one, that your Father also who is in the heavens may forgive you your trespasses;*
>
> *and, if ye do not forgive, neither will your Father who is in the heavens forgive your trespasses.'* (YLT) (Note added.)

Why insert admonishment to forgive right in the middle of a teaching on the power of our spoken word? Souls carrying unforgiveness are, apparently, without the power and authority God wants us to wield. I know my soul was.

"On Earth as In Heaven" is an Actual Goal

I believe that the "body of Christ" can slam the door on cancer (or any enemy lie) and lock that door. I believe that Jesus taught a particular prayer for a reason. Again, let's look at Matthew 6:10: *Our Father Who art in heaven. Hallowed be thy name. Thy Kingdom come. Thy will be done on earth as in heaven . . .* (KJV)

Again, there is NO disease in heaven. There should be no disease on earth. When we "do this truth"; we will be the "spotless Bride" of our Lord. Right now we are believing that all of our circumstances are bound up in the realm we "see" only **after** the fact. We can "see" **before** the fact, and, in doing so, we change what we see "in fact".

Like the Centurion, the woman with the blood issue, or other participants in Jesus's miracles, we must understand that our interaction in our own miracles is primarily our intent. Jesus called it *"faith"* and the writer of Hebrews called it *"the substance of things hoped for"*. If we have a disease, what is the *"thing hoped for"*? It is health! What can make it appear? Well, God spoke the entire universe into existence (Hebrews 11:3.) He was the "observer" and the "energy of His words" made it appear as He spoke it. We are created in His image (Genesis 1:27). We are creative beings with the power of intent within our thoughts and words. Jesus said so.

Why would a person diagnosed with cancer put their name on a prayer list? Who would they want to intercede for them? I don't know about you but I want intercessors with knowledge of *truth* not just sympathy regarding *facts*. I want people praying who intend for my healing to manifest as a result of their *compassionate* focus and intent As Rev. Cal Pierce says in *Healing, the Process to Divine Health,* "Sympathy locks you in and Compassion delivers you out." [7] Knowledge of truth opens the door for compassion.

Prophesy, Prayer, and The Speed of Light Coincide

David Van Koevering says it well: "Two thirds of your Bible got to mankind before the event or cause! All creativity comes before the actual reality! What is a vision? What is a word of knowledge? It is seeing, knowing, getting information before the causation. There is no other source of creativity than the Holy Spirit. All truth comes to man through the only source of truth we have and that is the Holy Spirit. When you see your future, you are getting information faster than the speed of light through a means of streaming superluminal (faster than light) particles. The barrier of light speed is bridged from this subluminal (slower than light) realm to the higher bandwidth of the superluminal realm by the Holy Spirit." [8]

I would add to Van Koevering's questions: "What is an idea?" and "What word will be spoken as a result of that 'idea'?" What is prophecy? What energy will be released by that word? When a person is praying for me, I want them to have the idea that my health is already a "done deal" because of Jesus' finished work and the inheritance He secured. I want them to **intend** for their word to accomplish a restoration of specific elements of my health. I do not want them pleading with God to do what He's already done. I want them commanding my body to function as God created it to function and still **intends** it to function until my days are fulfilled. I want them asking the Lord to show them how they need to pray to bring about specific manifestation of my health rather than asking IF it's His will for me to be healed. His Word (logos) already established His will.

Throughout cancer's attacks on my body, I could sense, even when unconscious, that there was a deliberate pulsating energy around and within me that was positive and creative. Since my recovery, I have been blessed to meet some of those who prayed for me including friends of my family members. I was also blessed that the people of Pastor Tom's church had been well taught how *"faith is the substance of things hoped for"* and sent that substantive energy toward me with intent. I was "receiving" that energy because I was not conscious. Pastor Tony Kemp (www.tonykempministries.net), a highly anointed healing minister, taught me that we cannot "send and receive" at the same time; so we should get quiet and focus on receiving when being prayed for. This teaching speaks to the power of our intent.

When I "got back on my feet" even tottering on a walker, the little bit of Scripture I knew was seed for more discovery. My thoughts had to be creative and I had to take God at His creative word. I am going to refer to Gary Sinclair as I finish this chapter praying that my reader will grab hold of the power available to them for locking cancer and other disease out of their lives.

Sinclair, whose counseling ministry is "Celebrate Live", says he has counseled many people who have been taught a counterfeit version of the spiritual lessons within Quantum Mechanics. I, too, observe that Christians have let the enemy co-opt much of the knowledge in Quantum Mechanics by ignoring its convergence with Scripture. They forget that the powerless enemy must corrupt our perception of those things that empower us. We should not take the bait to ignore the science God created. Some modern movements that delve into Quantum Mechanics are all dressed up in philosophical trappings and teach such things as "you are God" - sometimes on the programs of very popular television personalities.

Sinclair says that he has worked with many people who have been taught this lie in certain movements only to become terribly frustrated at their own powerlessness. Pondering his clients' frustration with being taught "they are God", Sinclair shares that "we recognize God as Omnipresent and yet still create our individual identity of separateness" . . . "There is only one gift that God made each of us individually responsible for. That gift is *thought*. Some have called it a free will gift. When you recognize that God promised never to violate your free will, you will realize the immense value He placed on your ability to use this gift of thought." [9]

Sinclair harkens back to Dr. Candace Pert's *Molecules of Emotion* saying, "You sow in *seed thought* that which you wish to reap in harvest . . . Thus, the only way to change your conditions in life is to change your thoughts about life. The road to health begins in your secret thoughts and the motivating power that keeps it coming is your constructive energizing emotions staying focused on the outcome."[10]

We have used Sinclair's term "inter-active miracles" throughout this book. He writes, "At the level of desire, you create the seeds of miracles . . . for God in His faithfulness has promised you the *desires of your heart*." (Psalms 37:4) [11]

Let us stand on our foundation regarding intent as we look at the power of words and thoughts regarding health.

seven

Using the Power of Words

U nder the threatening diagnosis of cancer, thoughts and images often torment. Every discouraging medical term or pitiful glance can heighten fears and raise anxiety. Keeping a cool head throughout the process of slamming the door on cancer helps cool down the process of dis-ease within the body. In fact, every belief and every word spoken over ourselves is powerful. The ability to step into the beautiful life involves harnessing the power of every thought to choose life and dis-empower death.

I shared scientist Masuru Emoto's illustration of the power of intent in the last chapter; however, Emoto also demonstrated in his laboratory that words actually change matter. His work is evocative regarding healing considering that our bodies are more than 70% water. Emoto used special microscopic cameras to photograph crystals from water exposed to written or spoken words. From words like "you fool" and "satan", he obtained horribly misshapen crystals. The most symmetrical and beautiful crystals came from water exposed to the words "gratitude" and "love" in that order. [1]

This experiment would not be news to the Apostle Paul who surely recognized the innate role of gratitude within our organic balance as he wrote to the Ephesians: ...*speaking to yourselves in psalms and hymns and spiritual songs, singing and making melody in your heart to the Lord, giving thanks always for all things, in the name of our Lord Jesus Christ, to the God and Father.* (Ephesians 5:19-20, YLT)

We have seen that Scripture and science converge in recognizing the soul-body healing continuum. This convergence adds to our further discussion of the impact our words have on our health. Rev. Henry W. Wright says, "Science is man understanding what has always been." He points out that, "Without recognizing the spirit world, science is defective". He also says that many "Spiritual Leaders" don't understand this fact any better than scientists do because neither actually studies the Word of God deeply enough. [2]

The substance of Wright's remarks have been reflected in my own research which compelled me to discuss the topics in this book from both a Spiritual and scientific perspective including the following overview of the power of words and thoughts. We will also discuss the wonderful power of decreeing Scriptures or God's word into our very beings. We have seen Quantum Physics recently opening up exciting ways we can impact our own health. I want to share a very interesting exercise. Think of thoughts as the quantum level of "body-mind" just like electrons are quantum level of electricity and photons are quantum level of light.[3]

In my seminars I do a demonstration learned from Gary Sinclair. I ask for a volunteer who is physically strong to come forward. Then I ask him/her to say aloud ten times, "I am worthy and strong". When they finish, I have them extend their dominant arm out to the side parallel to the floor and I try to push down on their arm. It's always difficult and usually impossible to push the arm down even though I am quite strong now. I follow this "test" by asking them to envision a **fictional** person standing a few feet away from them. I ask if it is a man or woman to make sure they have a specific fabrication. Then I have them repeat ten times aloud, "**You** are unworthy and weak." Once they complete the repetitions, I have them extend the same arm in the same way and I try to push it down just as before. ALWAYS, I have been able to push the arm down easily with hardly any resistance. It is amazing, but their body has believed what they just repeated to a person who doesn't even exist while they were fully aware it was untrue.

There are both spiritual and scientific dynamics at work in responding to our own words and those spoken to us. The demonstration I just shared indicates that words dramatically impact our bodies, but why are they so important? Obviously, words are first formed as either positive or negative thoughts. When spoken, the words give "life" to the root thought either by causing an action or by causing more thoughts. Later, we examine this concept further with the help of Dr. Caroline Leaf, PhD, a brilliant Christian psychologist.

Dr. David Younggi Cho, pastor of the largest Christian church in the world, devotes a full chapter of his book, *The Fourth Dimension*, to the power of words. He describes having breakfast with one of Korea's leading neurosurgeons who asked, 'Dr. Cho, did you know that the speech center in the brain rules over all the nerves?' You ministers really have power, because, according to our recent findings in neurology, **the speech center in the brain has total dominion over all the other nerves.**"[4]

Cho says he laughed and told the physician "I've known that for a long time . . . I learned it from 'Dr. James' . . . He was one of the famous doctors in Biblical times . . . and, in his book, chapter three, the first few verses clearly defines the activity and importance of the tongue and the speech center." The neurosurgeon continued, "The speech nerve center has such power over all of the body that simply speaking can give one control over his body, to manipulate it in the way he wishes. He said, 'If someone keeps on saying, "I'm going to become weak,' then right away, all the nerves receive that message, and they say, 'Oh, let's prepare to become weak, for we've received instructions from our central communication that we should become weak'. They then, in natural sequence, adjust their physical attitudes to weakness." [5]

Cho shares several more examples the physician gave him; however, let's look at what the Biblical, "Dr. James" said using "the tongue" to indicate "speech" in James 3:5-11:

> Likewise the **tongue** is a small part of the body, but it makes great boasts. Consider what a great forest is set on fire by a small spark. The **tongue** also is a fire, a world of evil among the parts of the body. It corrupts the whole person, sets the whole course of his life on fire, and is itself set on fire by hell.
> All kinds of animals, birds, reptiles and creatures of the sea are being tamed and have been tamed by man,
> but no man can tame the **tongue**. It is a restless evil, full of deadly poison.
> With the **tongue** we praise our Lord and Father, and with it we curse men, who have been made in God's likeness.
> Out of the same **mouth** come praise and cursing. My brothers, this should not be.
> Can both fresh water and salt water flow from the same spring? (NIV)

When Our Words Match God's Words, Good Happens

Both Annette Capps and her father, Charles Capps, a very insightful minister and author, have strongly ministered to me in my overcoming pancreatic cancer. If I had to choose a single resource to credit as my "Number Two Tool" after the Bible itself, it would be Charles Capps' small but rich book, *God's Creative Power*. I use it every single day and I have given away dozens of these books to people dealing with health issues.

This book is not a "name it and claim it" perversion of Scripture. It is solidly set in Scripture and teaches what Jesus taught. Charles Capps says, "Jesus always spoke the end results and not the problem. Never did He confess present circumstances. He spoke the desired results." [6] Capps continues about Jesus's praying: "He spent much time in prayer, but He never prayed the problem; He prayed the answer – **what God said is the answer.** He used the written Word (of God) to defeat Satan." [7]

Jesus, the "Word made Flesh" knew what the patriarchs had taught, like His earthly ancestor, the wise King Solomon. We see, here, reference to body and soul being affected by God's Words when we keep them in view: Proverbs 4:20-26 instructs:

> *My son, attend to my* **words***; consent and submit to my sayings.*
> *Let them not depart from your sight; keep them in the center of*
> *your heart.*
> *For they are* **life** *to those who find them,* **healing and health to**
> **all their flesh.**
> *Keep and* **guard your heart** *(soul) with all vigilance and above*
> *all that you guard, for out of it flow the springs of life.*
> *Put away from you false and dishonest speech, and willful and*
> *contrary talk put far from you.*
> *Let your eyes look right on [with fixed purpose], and let your gaze*
> *be straight before you.*
> *Consider well the path of your feet, and let all your ways be estab-*
> *lished and ordered aright.*

My own testimony includes a very critical and specific experience with "The Word". The first two years after my "strike two" cancer surgery, I went twice yearly for scans and blood work. Because I knew that I knew that I knew in my heart that cancer was behind me, I didn't really want to go; however, I was confident God was protecting me from the potential radiation damage of these tests - the kind of protection promised in Mark 16:18. I had prayed to be an encourager to others and felt I needed my healing to be well documented for that purpose.

About two weeks before I was scheduled for a routine screening, virtually **all** my symptoms returned with a vengeance. They were very specific and included such things as blood pressure fluctuating like a yo-yo; sudden onset dizziness, flushing, etc. I had a choice. I could choose what the enemy of my soul clearly "pushed" with toxic thoughts like "It's baaaack" and give in to fear or I could "take that thought captive" per Scripture as Paul writes in 2 Corinthians 10:5: *We demolish arguments* *and every pretension that sets itself up against the knowledge of God, and* **we take captive every thought to make it obedient to Christ.** (NIV)

I understood that I needed to DO more than deny symptoms. That would have been silly. I had real symptoms. The "woman with the issue of blood" whom we earlier studied had already defined a pattern for me in my inter-active miracle. Like her, I **spoke** into my atmosphere saying "I will go to the Lord and I will assure my healing once and for all."

I have since learned from Pastor Bill Johnson, that *"taking every thought captive" (2 Corinthians 10:5)* is to recognize a "worldly thought" or a thought bound by how the world considers circumstances and, once you have recognized it, to intentionally replace it with a "Kingdom thought" or a thought that agrees with the laws of Creation. [8] I have also come to realize, as earlier discussed, that sin is essentially denying the laws (principles) of Creation - laws that extend throughout both natural and spiritual law. Conversely, faith is a matter of ever increasing spiritual bandwidth and it brings insight, perspective, and discernment we cannot otherwise employ.

The enemy of our souls has no authority in this world but he does have power **IF and only IF** he can dominate human thoughts. I needed this truth at the point of severe symptomatic attack (facts) and God gave me yet another "just in time" mechanism. I had recently begun reading Charles Capps' book, *God's Creative Power*. Additionally, a church family that absolutely believed in God's Word regarding healing supported me. I had only positive energy working for me in the face of this attack.

Capps explains, "God's Word ministers to the total man. His Word (Jesus Himself) is our wisdom, righteousness, sanctification, and redemption." [9] This decree led me to remember that "healing IS a done deal" as Jesus's own words from the cross emphasize: *"It is finished!* (John 19:30). The cross and resurrection left nothing still to be done except for all people to realize the full impact of that event. I screamed at the enemy, "You are toast! I am fully aware that Jesus finished you!" Then, realizing that Jesus used the "Sword of the Spirit" or Word of God to defuse the enemy's bullying in his wilderness test, I grabbed my copy of

God's Creative Power and began to read aloud (because the enemy cannot read our minds). I read every Scriptural decree in that book at least three times a day just like taking medicine. Three or four days went by and the enemy fired thoughts, "You aren't healed. You still have symptoms. You are going to have terrible test results. You just thought you could stand up and fight me."

But, like "the woman with the issue of blood", I became very focused and continued to decree the healing promises of God aloud. I told no one else of the symptoms. I just got alone and decreed the Scriptures. The words became engrafted into my body and soul through my attention/ intention and the vibration of Scripture read aloud. Within 5 days, all the symptoms were totally gone and the tests and scans I underwent the next week were absolutely perfect like they had been previous times and have remained. The underlying principle at work here is "calling things that are not as though they are" which is exactly the way God spoke the universe into being. Again, I was NOT denying what was. Doing so is negative and silly. I was cooperating with the universal law of creation. Doing that is positive and powerful. The vibrations of my own flesh came into resonance with the vibrations of God's Word, which expresses His intention.

I am not recommending that others keep symptoms a secret. In my case I knew I would overcome the attack and I did not want to alarm my loved ones. Nor did I want to chance a single doubt being spoken into the situation - NO sympathy! I was already scheduled for scans in two weeks so I began to focus on reports of scan results by continuing to decree, "no evidence of residual or recurrent disease" rather than giving fear an opening.

I still read these Scriptural decrees once daily. It's not bondage or ritual for me; it is a means of connecting with Health – God Himself. I repeat, "Your body is listening to you and it will obey you. Charles Capps agrees with Pastor Chou's neurosurgeon, "The part of the body (brain) that controls speech also controls chemical secretion to the body. This sheds considerable light on Jesus's words in Mark 11:23: ". . . *he shall have whatsoever he **says**.*" [10]

Kenneth E. Hagin, whose teaching emits faith, was a teen-ager near death, paralyzed and suffering with a cardiac birth defect when he discovered Mark 11:23 in his grandmother's Bible. He believed it, applied it with the persistent fervor of David going at Goliath, and became completely healed. I highly recommend Hagin's workbook, *Healing Bible Study Course*. I believe the teachings of both Hagin and Capps are extraordinarily practical.

Words emit either fear or faith but never both. No good thing ever arises from fear. Think of the impact of such clichés` as "That just burns me up." "I'm scared to death.", "I'm trying to get the flu." or "This headache is killing me." As Capps says, "The truth is, your body always responds to your words in some manner, either for better or worse. So choose your words carefully." [11]

Pastor Anita Siddiki, of Wisdom Ministries, tells a profound story about her mother who loved the Lord and was one of the most faithful saints in her church. When, she was diagnosed with cancer it much perplexed her church family because of the "beautiful life" she lived. Although they prayed for her and her healing manifested once, she eventually died from the disease. Anita shares that she had accompanied her mother on home visits to the elderly many times (before cancer) and, consistently upon leaving a home, her mother would say, "Anita, I don't ever want to grow old like that." Apparently, her body listened to her words. This wonderful woman, according to her daughter, never really contended for her healing from cancer.[12]

We often wonder why people we pray for do not see their healing manifest, but we may be totally unaware of the words they are speaking over themselves. Unfortunately, loved ones sometimes unknowingly speak words over their friends or family members that may undermine healing. I have seen people stop a friend, for example, in a cafe to ask about a family member's "battle with cancer". Often, the encounter becomes a litany of sympathetic phrases such as:

Well-meaning friend: "Say, Joe, how is your brother, Bob, doing? I saw him on the church prayer list."

Joe: "Well, he's really weak and tired. He said his last chemo treatment nearly killed him. He can't eat anything and he's on a lot of pain medication. All we can do is pray."

Well-meaning friend: "I'm sorry to hear that, but I'm glad they are at least taking care of his pain. We'll keep Bob in our prayers. Keep the faith!"

What kind of energy do these words emit? Does this conversation focus on the enemy's work or God's Word? I'm compelled to ask, "Keep what faith?" I mean no criticism regarding such dialogue - please just focus on the point at hand, which is that our words can unknowingly agree with the enemy, which, in turn, empowers him. We avoid this error by knowing what God says about healing and sharing it just like the fencing contractor did with me. Testimonies are power!

I once visited a church where the minister was going over the prayer list and announced that a certain member dealing with cancer "is actually feeling pretty well right now but we need to keep praying because we know it can't last." Again, my intent is not criticism but illustration of the subtle ways the enemy sneaks into our circumstances through ill-considered words and misplaced sympathy. I couldn't help but think of the "pity seeds" sewn in those who were likely to visit this church member who really needed positive encouragement and compassion rather than sympathy.

God's Word is Never a "Last Resort"

Dodie Osteen, in her book, *Healed of Cancer,* shares her own testimony of overcoming metastatic liver cancer after doctors gave her just a few months to live in 1981. Without surgery, chemotherapy or radiation, Dodie is healthy over 30 years later and still actively encouraging others. A registered nurse and then well known pastor's wife and now a nationally known pastor's mother, Dodie shares some words she habitually spoke **prior to her illness** saying, "I remember, when somebody would ask, 'How are you?' I would reply, 'I am disgustingly healthy!' After cancer came upon my body, I realized how foolish those words were'." [3] Our bodies believe **every** word we say.

Mrs. Osteen also shares how her family helped her escape the insidious grasp of self-pity, even though her healing manifested slowly, saying, "My children treated me as if I were a normal healthy mother. From the time John (her husband) and I prayed, they believed that I was healed. Sometimes there were things in the house that needed to be done, which I would ask them to do. But because they believed I was healed, they insisted that I could do them. It is a good thing they treated me as if I were healed; otherwise, many times I would have been tempted to have pity parties. They would not allow me to feel sorry for myself. They reminded me of the Word of God and of the prayer of faith we had prayed . . . Don't sit around and feel sorry for yourself when you are fighting the battle for your healing. Pity never wins! I overcame my pity parties by speaking to my body and commanding it to come in line with the Word of God. And it did!" [14] I also much admired the fact that Mrs. Osteen got outside her home and ministered to others as soon as she possibly could, and she shares how doing so strengthened her.

Finally, our discussion of the impact of words must include the 'Nocebo Effect" and "Placebo Effect" noted in medical literature. Without delving too deeply into the abundant literature on both subjects, I must mention that these word based "effects" are well-documented illustrations of the power of other people's words directly impacting healing. The "Placebo Effect" refers to the "healing" induced in patients participating in pharmaceutical clinical trials who are told they are being given an effective new drug although they are actually receiving inert "doses of the medicine". The "Nocebo Effect" refers to the many documented "deaths on schedule" of people who have been told by experts that they have a specific length of time to live. Some of them actually being "cancer free" when they died "on schedule". Our bodies don't merely listen to words, but they obey them.

"Words We Think" Impact our Health

I earlier referred to the work of Dr. Caroline Leaf, PhD, believer in Christ, researcher and highly respected psychologist. She has done groundbreaking work on how our brains process words and thoughts. I find her particularly discerning because she deals with more than facts such as anatomical structures by insightfully relating the science to Scripture. We know from scientific fact and spiritual truth that an unhealed soul blocks healing, and, I believe, that truth or "law" is particularly important in cancer even though Scripture assures us that "every disease" was covered through Jesus's finished work. (See Matthew 4:23 and 9:35.)

Let's examine Dr. Leaf's teaching on the power of our minds where stress from words, thoughts, and emotions enter. In her book, *Who Switched Off My Brain?* Leaf teaches that there are three stages of stress: temporary stress, unreleased stress (temporary that begins to become harmful), and finally, chronic stress. [15]

"When you are in chronic stress. your systems reach exhaustion from the constant state of heightened alert."[16] We earlier mentioned that a prolonged defensive or emergency mode is really a sustained inflammatory response? From my own reading, I believe chronic stress is comparable to "a sustained inflammatory response". Dr. Leaf, explaining from a psychological viewpoint, continues, "These stages of stress are scientifically significant because they illustrate how a single toxic thought causes extreme reactions in so many of our systems."[17]

Dr. Leaf states pointedly, "You must confront repressed unforgiveness, anger, rage, hatred or any other form of toxic thinking. **You have a medical need to forgive others and you also must forgive yourself.**"[18] She goes on to explain that stress resulting from our allowing toxic thoughts to linger and recycle in our minds have particularly detrimental effects on our hearts, our **immune systems**, and our digestive systems."[19] It is a consistent Biblical lesson that we should not worry or fear. Paul states is plainly: ... *for God did not give us a spirit of fear, but of power, and of love, and of a sound mind.* (2 Timothy 1:7, YLT)

Likewise, it's a consistent theme in this book that Spiritual or supernatural law is a continuum of science or natural law. Quantum science is fast revealing this truth so that sometimes we glimpse the science behind the miraculous. David Van Koevering's statement that the Spiritual (supernatural) is a widening "bandwidth" of the natural that I shared earlier is, I believe, much more than a metaphor. I observe that Van Koevering, in his bandwidth analogy, is expressing much the same insight as 19th century scientist/theologian I referenced earlier, Henry Drummond, who intimated that natural law illustrates spiritual law when he said, "I discovered myself enunciating Spiritual Law in the exact terms of Biology and Physics. Now this was not simply a scientific coloring given to Religion, the mere freshening of the theological air with natural facts and illustrations. It was an entire recasting of truth. . I saw. . that it meant essentially the introduction of Natural Law into the Spiritual World."[20] Jesus used parables to make this introduction.

In this same vein of thought, referring to John 16:13 (below), David Van Koevering goes so far as to conclude, "Jesus told His disciples that they will get their **upper** bandwidth back . . . *He* adds, "Jesus is saying, 'I want to show you your future. You can know my will and my plan for your life, although right now, you don't have the upper bandwidth to see or observe it."[21]

> *I have yet many things to say unto you, but ye cannot bear them now.*
> *Howbeit when he, the Spirit of truth, is come, he shall guide you into all the truth: for he shall not speak from himself; but what things soever he shall hear, these shall he speak: and he shall declare unto you the things that are to come.* (John 16:12-13, ASV)

We know that Holy Spirit arrived at Pentecost and remains within Believers who accept Him.

Could the Apostle Paul have been telling us that, as we in God's earthly Kingdom grow into His Love through our ever widening Spiritual bandwidth, we will eventually move into "His Kingdom coming on earth as in heaven" when he wrote 1 Corinthians 13:12-13: *For we see now through a mirror obscurely, and then face to face; now I know in part, and then I shall fully know, as also I was known; and now there doth remain faith, hope, love– these three; and the greatest of these is love.* (YLT)

These verses close the famous "love chapter" and I urge you to read all of I Corinthians 13 as soon as possible praying for divine insight.

Dr. Caroline Leaf masterfully joins truth and fact (Spiritual and natural law) as she teaches, "Even though you can't always control your circumstances, you can make fundamental choices that will help you control your reaction to your circumstances and keep toxic input out of your brain." [22]

"If you change your attitude and determine to apply God's excellent advice not to worry, the hypothalamus will cause the secretion of chemicals that facilitate the feeling of peace, and the rest of the brain will respond by secreting the correct "formula" of neurotransmitters for thought building and clear thinking."[23] You may recall that "molecules of emotion" that have receptors on every body cell are neurotransmitters.

The process Dr. Leaf describes for accomplishing this "peace" is a virtual "how to" for "taking every thought captive" which, to me, has been one of the Bible's most helpful teachings for soul healing in 2 Corinthians 10:5: *We demolish arguments and every pretension that sets itself up against the knowledge of God, and we **take captive every thought** to make it obedient to Christ.* (NIV)

What does it mean scientifically to act upon this Scriptural advice the Apostle Paul wrote to the strong willed early Corinthian Church? Dr. Leaf says that thoughts or "incoming information" are first in a "temporary state". "It (the thought) has not yet lodged itself into your memory or become a part of your spirit which defines who you are. You can choose to reject the presently activated thoughts and the incoming information, or you can let the information make its way into your mind (your soul) and your spirit, eventually subsiding to your non-conscious, which dominates who you are. [24]

Dr. Leaf stresses that we must make a conscious decision to accept or reject allowing a thought to move past temporary status.

Kenneth E. Hagin used a humorous but memorable metaphor for making the decision just described. He is often quoted as saying, "You can't keep a bird from flying around your head, but you can keep it from building a nest in your hair." This metaphor has "checked" me many times in my effort to make sure a toxic thought is temporary. Sometimes I say out loud, "No! I will not think that way. Forget It!" My goal is zero tolerance for "re-cycling negative thought energy".

Why? Because, as Dr. Leaf, eloquently points out, "As we start to understand how a thought forms and impacts our emotions and bodies, we have two choices: We can let our thoughts become toxic and poisonous, or we can detox our negative thoughts which will improve our emotional wholeness and even recover our physical health." [25] I hope you are realizing the unavoidable connection between thoughts, words, and soul wounds as blocks to physical healing. Dr. Leaf's book is a handbook for taking every thought captive. It's no wonder that Jesus put such strong emphasis upon wholeness in His ministry.

I love the Biblical story of Jonah in the belly of the fish. Most people have heard it. I would say that his circumstances were pretty bleak; however, he took every thought captive and scoffed at them as written in Jonah 2:8: *Those observing* **lying vanities** *their own mercy forsake.* (YLT)

Instead of "lying vanities" other translations call these thoughts "**vane imaginations**". We all know we can let our imaginations go wild "snowballing" a toxic worry.

Meditation– To Empty or to Fill, That is the Question

In my eighteen or so months between "strike one" and "strike two", I was aware that God had heard my foxhole prayer during the CT Scan that revealed the nature of my first tumor. However, I had such a weak foundation in God's Word that I didn't understand its power. It wasn't until my relapse brought me to church for my "oil service" and kept me there that I got my revelation: "The Bible is true". So, "between strikes", my seeking was random with my not realizing that some of it actually flirted with "man-made religions". I had a casual "friend" who insisted via email that I needed to learn to meditate. I did try it, but I found "emptying the mind" fruitless. Then what? And worse, "guided imagery" with meeting a contrived "healer" in an" imagined place" seemed ridiculous– how do you trust a contrived stranger?

Thank God, I was strongly compelled to read Psalms during this time, and, in them, David's meditating on all God had done for him and his people began to resonate in my soul. David, "a man after God's own heart" (See 1 Samuel 13:14 and Acts 13:22), actually talks to his own soul often in Psalms and his doing so inspired me. He modeled asking one's own soul what is troubling it fully expecting his relationship with God to inspire resolution. Reading Psalms made "emptying the mind" meditation as absurd to me as trying to fuel my body by emptying my stomach.

Now that I understand through quantum physics that meditating on the living Word of God actually physically resonates in my body, soul and spirit, I like that it puts THE Sword of THE Spirit in my hand - the same weapon that David used to be-head the bully, Goliath and that Jesus used to silence satan in the wilderness.

Obviously, God values our whole being - body, soul, and spirit. The religious doctrine that the "flesh" is bad, I believe, insults the atoning work of Christ Jesus, a work that obviously includes sacrifice for body, soul, and spirit. Allow me to point out a helpful correction. Hebrews 4:12 says: . . . *for the reckoning (word) of God is living, and working, and sharp above every two-edged sword, and piercing unto the dividing asunder both of soul and spirit, of joints also and marrow, and a discerner of thoughts and intents of the heart.* (YLT)

I cite this literal translation because, according to Greek scholar/theologian/teacher Harold Eberle, many translations imply that the Word of God is a Sword separating spirit (good) from soul (bad) when the original language is clear that God's Word actually separates the good from the evil within both our spirit and soul. Eberle says, "It is soul and spirit being pierced through "removing anything (in both) that is not in line with the nature of God which is consistent with the rest of the Bible." [26]

I absolutely believe I would not be alive today without the life empowering experience of meditating on the living, breathing Word of God because it fills the mind and body with health itself, hope itself, faith itself, love itself. It is THE "Real Thing".

Section III

The Power of Your Body to Heal Itself

"Our bodies want to be well. There is an innate wisdom within all of life that knows how to fix disease. No one has to tell the scab on your hand how to heal properly. You body knows what to do. We just have to give our body the proper physical and metaphysical resources to do its job right while purging our systems of toxins that inhibit healing."

Patrick Quillen, PhD in *Beating Cancer With Nutrition*

eight

Loving Your Body to Life

God, the Creator of heaven and earth created each of us. He knows you inside and out. And he has a specific plan for your life including body, soul and spirit. His protocol for health and restoration is so individual that I cannot give you a prescription for you to treat your body. There is no one size fits all plan for slamming the door on cancer because you are unique. It is up to you to listen for the Word and the plan that God gives to you. I hope, as you read this book, you are realizing what you need to do to work through emotional issues that facilitate dis-ease and coming into a new understanding of the power of God's word and the words you speak over yourself that facilitate divine health. Embrace the love of God and embrace your capability to love yourself and your body into wholeness. It is time to love your body into life.

We live in an "instant society" expecting to push a button and get desired results. Consequently, we might prefer a "smart phone app" to sustain our health. Certainly instantaneous miracles do occur, and, occasionally, the healing includes overt sensation. Generally, we must move into our healing through faith. And faith requires that we receive God's love for us and for ourselves. God loves you and me enough to tell us what we each need. Do you love yourself enough to follow though?

Spend a little time Scripturally walking with Jesus and you will notice that He moves in the "natural" and the "spiritual or supernatural" simultaneously. Earlier I mentioned, Pastor Anita Siddiki sharing the impact of words upon her precious mother's health. Anita, herself, is totally recovered from blindness and paralysis due to MS, which required great persistence mentally, physically and spiritually. Her husband, Nasir, discouraged other well-meaning family members from bringing her a wheel chair. The Siddiki's played tapes of Healing Scriptures 24/7 at Anita's bedside. And Anita shares that God also "downloaded" to her certain "natural instructions" like foods her body needed. [1] I believe Anita's testimony agrees with our premise in this book that we must tune into God and He will tell us what to do in our life to overcome, indeed slam the door on, diseases including but not limited to cancer.

There are hundreds of "one size fits all" healing protocol books and many make some good points, BUT I again urge you to begin with prayer for direction by first asking God to direct you to pertinent Scripture. Pray fervently as we've discussed, wait for God's movement in your spirit, confirm that it IS God's voice, then act upon His guidance which may include both "natural action" perhaps including some specific help from medical science as well as "spiritual action". Always ask Him to show you if there is someone you must forgive. Sometimes people focusing on spiritual aspects of healing will ignore directions God is giving them regarding everyday life including food, sleep, etc. My own restoration of health has included a great deal of change in both natural and spiritual lifestyle but my exact story will not perfectly overlay anyone else's. I am sharing it for encouragement and illustration. I've heard Pastor Bill Johnson say, "There are times God is looking for a celebration response to natural processes as well as supernatural". [2]

Jesus Moved in Both the "Natural" and the "Supernatural"

Jesus modeled interactive miracles repeatedly.

Jairus, a synagogue leader, came to Jesus asking Him to come heal his little daughter. Jesus actually raises the child from death following with absolutely "natural" instructions in Luke 8:50-56: *And her spirit returned [from death], and she arose immediately; and He directed that she should be given something to eat.*

Jesus does something quite "supernatural" one moment and quite "natural" the next. The girl is "in life", indeed, in "health again" and that status requires eating food.

Jesus gives authority to his disciples in Mark 6: 12,13 and then Mark 6:30-32, and sends them out to into neighboring villages to drive out unclean spirits and heal the sick. He tells them to take no provisions except a walking stick – no money, no food, etc. But in the later verses the disciples return and tell Jesus amazing miracles they accomplished supernaturally. Jesus then suggests they find a deserted place and get some rest and nourishment. They were working miracles one day; yet resting and eating natural food the next.

In Matthew 15:32-39, Jesus has been teaching a large crowd for three days when the disciples come saying there is nothing left to eat. Instead of just miraculously making all these people "no longer physically hungry", He has the disciples gather what little food is left, gives thanks asking the Father God to bless it, and in complete faith, hands out the multiplied provisions so that thousands of people can get their bellies full of natural food.

As you read Scripture, watch for the many examples of Jesus moving at once in the natural and supernatural. We must as well and be ever alert to each bit of improvement experienced being sure to express our gratitude and praise. That expression, itself, is tremendously empowering as is watching for our healing rather than our disease symptoms.

Even in the natural anti-cancer lifestyle elements we are about to consider, I can only share what I have discovered and found helpful. My blogs also offer additional resources with hundreds of posts sorted by topics and dates. Information is essential, but staying tuned into God's perfect plan for each of us is primary.

Ways to Love your Body to Life

I have mentioned that "insult" or trauma triggers inflammatory responses. This reaction can occur for a variety of possible reasons including repeated "insult" that becomes chronic rather than subsiding after completing its "regular job" within the healing process. If the "insult" persists, the chronic inflammation can localize leading to tumorous growth (see Appendix Five).

Remember the analogy of our cells being like fish in an aquarium? We need to filter body fluid (lymph) to overcome our diseased and dirty inner terrain where our cells must live. How do we do so?

First, we must end the stimulating "insult" that sends inflammatory chemicals into the blood stream making capillary walls super porous. Then we must get the extra fluid and debris out of the space between the cells. That job falls to the under-appreciated lymph vessels paralleling the blood vessels throughout body tissue. Unlike blood, lymph fluid has no heart-like "pump" moving it. And lymph moves slowly in only one direction requiring check valves to avoid backwash.

In that work, the lymph capillaries pick up fluid from body tissue and carry it to soda straw sized ducts. Nodes filter out toxins and debris. Then the fluid pours into a vein under the collarbone. To overcome "stagnation", we absolutely must keep that lymph fluid moving steadily, sometimes against gravity. How?

Draining the Swamp

Let's look at the important mechanisms we can use to help our lymphatic system do its critical job. I'll discuss each of these in more detail shortly.

Muscle contraction all over the body "squeeze pumps" lymph capillaries and helps move lymph fluid out of body tissue.

Deep Breathing is a mechanism shown to expedite lymph movement.

Laughter has proven to be "the best medicine" as Scripture and science both teach, and one reason is that it is mechanically helpful in moving lymph.

Lymphatic Massage can be helpful in facilitating lymph fluid movement, but should be done by trained technicians to avoid damage to superficial nodes.

Beneficial Ways to Exercise

I am providing information regarding exercises known to help stimulate lymph movement. Making exercise decisions is another area to pray about as we have discussed. I used to think we shouldn't bother God with such things. I was absolutely wrong. He cares about every thing we care about. Timing may be important and it is an individual matter.

Movement Routine: We need to exercise in ways that intermittently compress and relax tissues from the movement as well as using deep breathing patterns. Think of the lymph system as being a bit like a tree with roots, a trunk, and branches. The arms, shoulders, head and neck are the branches and the legs are the roots with the trunk actually being in our "trunk". I use an exercise routine I adapted from some 'Tai Chi like" movements. Just go to YouTube and search "Slam the Door on Cancer Exercise Video". In this exercise routine, I deliberately breathe in when moving limbs toward my body trunk and breath out when moving limbs away from my body trunk.

Bouncing on a Mini-trampoline is a popular enjoyable way to "lymphasize" body tissue. When I am bouncing, I deliberately breathe aggressively and rhythmically in through nose and out through mouth and often hold 4 lb. hand weights that I move in ways targeting certain muscle groups. I lost considerable muscle mass after so many surgeries. With my smaller pancreas, I felt I needed to avoid insulin resistance so I deliberately built back my muscle cells through exercise, and, thereby, gained insulin receptors on those cells. I have never supplemented insulin because my goal is not changing lab results but maintaining "the healthy state". My regular blood tests remain perfect.

Swimming is another "lymphasizing" exercise I enjoy varying my routine. One benefit of the water exercising is to have the external water pressure against body tissue "massaging" any pockets of "inflammation" trapped by surgical scar tissue while incurring beneficial muscle contraction against water resistance. Dr. Harvey Bigelsen, MD, discusses trapped post surgery inflammation at length in his book *Doctors are More Harmful Than Germs*.

Dancing is my all time favorite exercise. I'm an artist (and you are too). I love painting while moving to music. It's fun to "dance through a painting". Moving music recorded with loving intention has specific healing resonances within it. Just put on some wholesome music and move. Singing is great too. I love dancing to the praise/worship music of Julie Meyer, Vince Gibson, Joann McFatter, Travis Cottrell, and Michael W. Smith among others.

Don't Forget the Whimsical

I'm compelled to add a note about "free" art and music in healing. You may not consider yourself an artist - but you are. I recommend you get a sketchbook and some markers or crayons and spend time doodling to music that will flow through your soul without calling attention to itself while it emits strong positive vibrations. Just move the crayon and get lost in it. Begin with no pre-conceived ideas and expect nothing . . . God will show up. You may "see" things in your "free play" paintings days later– images that help your soul heal.

If you ever played a musical instrument, maybe you could pick it back up . . . just for you. Or, you could get an inexpensive harmonica and learn a few tunes for fun. At least, get a kazoo but get two because someone else will want to join you. Breath deeply when you "play" and you are about to learn why. Try silly stuff like that and you will be amazed how healing it is. If the folks around you scoff at silliness, do it anyway. They aren't the bosses of you and, besides, fun is contagious. Get back to who "you" are by remembering "you" are not your body. You are a spirit with a soul living in a body. God is a fun God always in a good mood. When I learned to play and laugh with God, my healing took an actual "quantum leap".

Laughter is "Internal Jogging"

A rejoicing heart doth good to the body, And a smitten spirit dries the bone. (Proverbs 17:22, YLT)

We know that "rejoicing" can include a healing attitude of gratitude. Further, the Hebrew root for "gratitude" includes the words "joy and glee" which surely result in laughter. And the often-overlooked admonishment that *"a smitten spirit dries the bone"* points to moving body fluids around so that all tissue including the bones can be irrigated properly. Such irrigation would, of course, include the **bone marrow where stem cells originate for new body cells.** We are focused on replacing diseased cells with healthy cells, which means we need "joyfully irrigated" bone marrow. Science and Scripture fit hand in glove as this Proverb illustrates.

In his often quoted book, *Anatomy of an Illness,* Norman Cousins shares his testimony of using laughter therapy for overcoming a life threatening disease. He says, "What was significant about the laughter was not just the fact that it provides internal exercise for a person flat on his or her back– a form of jogging for the innards - but that it creates a mood in which the other positive emotions can be put to work too. In short, it helps make it possible for good things to happen." [3]

Henry W. Wright, in *A More Excellent Way to be in Health,* writes, "Do you know laughter can strengthen the immune system? It has been documented. Laughter causes the body to manufacture T cells and (natural) killer cells." [4] He concludes also: "The immune system is compromised because of fear and anxiety coming out of a broken heart." [5] This point is pertinent to our discussions of reaction to "insult".

I agree with Cousins and Wright. Cousins mentions watching videos of great comedy figures such as Charlie Chaplin and humorists such as Ogdon Nash and James Thurber. I enjoy Bill Cosby, Jeannie Robertson, Taylor Mason, Thor Ramsey, Michael Jr., Chonda Pierce, Anita Renfroe, et al available on digital media and YouTube. I urge you to "start laughing" now and begin to realize that your "inner swamp" is changing into a "cascade of vitality".

We know that our eyes (and ears) are "windows of our souls" so it is important to avoid media that transmits negative or "dark" energy into our atmosphere. For me, that includes minimizing exposure to news media and online social media. I've read that the average person today is exposed to more bad news in a day than they were in a year just five decades ago. I promise you there was plenty of bad news then, but media did not need to fill airwaves 24/7.

Healing Touch Is Important

Healing touch is another overlooked healing mechanism in our "digital society". Referring to followers of Christ, Jesus says, *they will lay their hands on the sick, and they will get well.* (Mark 16:18)

I can actually remember when physicians routinely touched patients to get a sense of their condition and impart healing. I can also remember lying in that ICU day after day and becoming aware of a loved one's touch. I needed their touch much more than another IV drip or CT scan. We know from science and Scripture how very important touch is because it is virtually transferring His power from within us. Again, Ephesians 3:20 reminds us: *Now to Him who is able to do immeasurably more than all we ask or imagine according to **His power that is at work WITHIN us**.*

Jesus touched anyone in need of healing including lepers, which I believe healed their souls wounded from the lonely isolation of their fear-ridden disease. Of course Jesus knew the power of the healing touch and, as mentioned earlier, admonished us to lay hands on the sick. (If you pray for someone, honor him or her by asking for their permission before laying hands on him or her.) Part of the James Chapter Five "oil service instructions" includes touch. We know, from new insights through quantum mechanics that all of creation is one indivisible dynamic whole in which energy and matter, as Einstein and others described, are so deeply entangled it is impossible to consider them as independent elements. [6]

Life processes ignoring this entanglement and the resulting need for loving interaction with each other break basic laws of Creation, and thus our souls are wounded making our bodies targets for "anti-life" forces which exist in the unseen realm (evil). A clear example of this wounding is documented in orphans who go without consistent loving touch in their lives.

What am I suggesting? Well, God is Love and Love heals! I remember a song, "Reach out and **touch** somebody's hand. Make this world a better place if you can." [7] It was sung over and over by the entire ceremony crowd at the 1984 Los Angeles Olympics. The positive impact of that moment was vibrant against the darkness of the boycott by several countries. Love always wins! Loving touch itself is powerful as Luke 6:19 shares: *The whole multitude sought to touch Him (Jesus) for power went out from Him and healed them all.*

That same Jesus is alive NOW. Mark 6:56 says: *I am He who lives, and was dead, and behold, I am alive forevermore.*

Romans 8:11 tells us: *If the Spirit of Him who raised Jesus from the dead* **dwells in you**, *He who raised Christ from the dead will also* **give life to your mortal bodies** *through* **His Spirit who dwells in you**.

Hugs, prayers with hands laid on, as well as warm handshakes emit positive healing energy when there is loving intent involved. We have mentioned the quantum power of intent throughout this book. Anyone who has ever fallen in love understands what I am talking about.

Holy Spirit's power is within us so we have, in our inheritance, a very real healing touch of pure energy enabling what we otherwise could never do. Hug your loved ones and you both will be positively energized. When you hug, place your heart over your loved ones heart with your heads facing over each other's left shoulders. I have read several places that doing so actually synchronizes the heartbeats of those who are hugging. Our bodily functions are electrical including our heartbeat. Shortly we will look at electrically charged nutrition and see the quantum basis for being "one" with God.

Cancer Hates "Sweet Sleep"

When you lie down, you will not be afraid; when you lie down, your sleep will be sweet. (Proverbs 3:24, NIV)

Sleep is overlooked in "cancer literature". Doctors will wake you up in the hospital for early morning rounds and then admonish you to "get plenty of sleep because we heal while sleeping". From my experience and research, attending to our sleep habits is essential for sustaining our body, soul and spirit in a "healthy state".

For a long time, scientists thought that only the brain needed to go "offline" and sleep. It is true that, when we run out of brain and nerve energy, we absolutely must sleep to revitalize it; however, these scientists overlooked that the body also needs to "go offline" and, thereby, heal and revitalize. We also know that sleep and dreaming are important to our soul and spirit in ways that implement "taking every thought captive".

Dr. Caroline Leaf's book, *Who Switched Off My Brain,* would be a concise "how to" reference for you on this point. We have already mentioned factors regarding toxic thoughts, which lead to worry, and then loss of the "sweet sleep" God's Word declares for us. Dr. Leaf says, "Quality and quantity of restful sleep are prerequisites for controlling toxic thoughts, emotions and body weight. When you sleep the brain sorts out your thinking for the next day and consolidates memories." [8]

In her book, *Rethinking Cancer,* Ruth Sackman says, "Not to give your body the sleep it wants is another **abuse of natural law** that can drain the vital life energies essential for overcoming disease."[9]

Every healthy body cell is equipped with two genes that stave off cancer - the "anti-oncogenes". As long as both are intact, the cell is protected, but if one or both are damaged, the cell is vulnerable to malignancy if its "environment" is defiled. Lack of deep sleep actually shuts down the activity of over 700 different genes, and, in particular, those controlling inflammation, immunity, stress, metabolism and cancer (directly and indirectly). "One thing is certain. Lack of DEEP sleep will shut off your DNA faster than most bad habits." [10]

Professor David Spiegel of Stanford University points out that how people sleep can seriously alter hormone balance in their bodies thereby influencing cancer progression. For example, cortisol, among many other hormones, regulates the immune system including Natural Killer cells - the enemy of cancer cells. Melatonin, which lowers estrogen, is another hormone affected by sleep. Some scientists believe diminished melatonin increases risk of cancer manifesting in the breast. [11]

Dr. William Dement, M.D., PhD, in his book, *The Promise of Sleep,* declares: "Whenever we fall asleep, the level of immune system molecules such as interleukin-1 and tumor necrosis factor (TNF) rise in the blood, then drop in the morning as we wake up. TNF is a potent killer of cancer. Dement adds: "Natural killer cells may be particularly affected by lack of sleep. Staying up all night doesn't appear to affect their levels during the sleepless night, but the next day the number of Natural Killer cells available to fight off invaders can be severely reduced. [12]

Dement also shares that sufficient and consistent deep sleep is critical for the body's ongoing cell repair and replacement. He also cited studies involving thousands of human subjects in which healthy longevity had a direct correlation to averaging eight hours of sleep per night and neither more or less.[13]

Deep Breathing vs. Cancer

Shortly we will discuss in more detail the result of oxygen being insufficiently supplied to body cells because the blocking of oxygen delivery to cells is within the cascade of events that push cells into malignancy. (See Appendix Five). Before we look at the science, I want to share a powerful oxygenation activity. Many people lead sedentary lives - habitually breathing shallow while body cells are gasping for oxygen.

I've heard stories of Indian tribes whose elders, when satisfied they had completed their lives, would go into the woods, sit quietly, purposely practice **shallow** breathing, and expire within 24 hours. This story makes physiological sense. Proper **deep** breathing is absolutely essential for healing and health. Without it, the lymphatic system absolutely cannot function optimally. On www.tomocklerpt.com, I found a very good deep breathing exercise demonstration that basically follows the steps I use listed below:

> **First,** place the tip of your tongue where your front teeth join gums.
> Apparently doing so completes an electrical circuit in the body.
> **Second,** focusing on filling your chest cavity, breath in through your nose to a comfortable count of four. Practice so you can gauge filling your lungs full to the count.

Third, hold that breath to a count of seven keeping the same pace as your inhale.

Fourth, keeping the tip of your tongue in place, expel your breath through your mouth making a "whoosh" sound to a count of eight staying with the same pace.

The count ratio is important because your heart beats several times per each breath phase accomplishing several critical functions including blood oxygenation and internal organ compression, which moves lymph fluid. The exhaling after holding a breath expels lymph fluid into the blood stream. There may be benefits to the body's electrical field as well because, as the lymph fluid (largely water) moves, a rebalance of the electrical fields occur. This ancient breathing practice has served me well. I recommend doing several breathing exercise sequences a day. I often do so waiting for traffic lights.

Fresh Oxygen and Positive Energy

Reflecting on quality of sleep and the importance of oxygen intake as well as the need to avoid toxic substances, I have found that keeping a nice assortment of green plants in my bedroom enhances the quality of my sleep and provides fresh oxygen in the air I breathe while sleeping and exercising which I also do there.

Houseplants can significantly help detoxify your home environment by either absorbing contaminants in leaf pores or by metabolizing contaminants through organisms living in the soil. Plants also help maintain humidity levels and remove mold spores and bacteria from the air. We know they release oxygen critical for preventing and overcoming cancer as we are about to examine further.

Here is a list of plants and the toxins they neutralize as reported on the often useful website of www.renegadehealth.com.

Spider Plant: formaldehyde, xylene and toluene.

Golden Pothos: benzene, formaldehyde, trichloroethylene, xylene and toluene.

Snake Plant (Mother-in-Law's Tongue): benzene, formaldehyde, trichloroethylene, xylene and toluene.

Bamboo Palm or Reed Palm: formaldehyde, xylene, and toluene.

Chinese Evergreen: benzene, formaldehyde.

Peace Lily: benzene, formaldehyde, trichloroethylene, xylene, toluene, and ammonia.

English Ivy: mold and mildew, formaldehyde, benzene, xylene, and toluene.

Gerbera Daisies: benzene, formaldehyde, trichloroethylene.

Red-Edged Dracaena (Dracaena Marginata): benzene, formaldehyde, trichloroethylene, xylene, and toluene.

Warneck Dracaena: benzene, trichloroethylene, xylene, and toluene.

Weeping Fig: formaldehyde, xylene, and toluene.

Chrysanthemum: formaldehyde, benzene, trichloroethylene, xylene, toluene, and ammonia.

Boston fern: formaldehyde, xylene and toluene.

Philodendron: formaldehyde. [14]

I believe living plants in my home contribute to the positive life force around me, which makes sense from what we are learning about vibrational exchange in matter through quantum mechanics.

Notes:

nine

Eat Sunshine

E at the sunshine! Bring light into your cells through what you eat and, in the process, discover fresh energy emerging as the healthy state of being returns.

Life at the cellular level is busy and we have already noted that a healthy cell will never get cancer and that our cells totally depend on what we send them to remain healthy. Cells deprived of efficient delivery of the oxygen and nutrients they need, indeed, that **we** need, kick into desperation mode and anaerobically ferment sugar to survive. Several health threats follow including interrupted normal life processes, acidity in body fluids, mineral imbalances, tumor formation, pain, energy depletion, and ultimately death. We have noted that physical and emotional "insults", if perpetuated, can hold us in a chronic inflammatory state forcing us into a sustained "defensive mode" in which we cannot create healthy new cells, as we must to live.

We can benefit from examining the related work of some brilliant scientists over the last century including Dr. Otto Warburg, Dr. Albert Einstein, and, again, Dr. Johanna Budwig. I personally find this information practical on a daily basis and believe it is an important part of my recovery and health maintenance. I share it to help you make choices. Please bear with me while we consider facts many people don't know about our body cells because we need to understand more about the place in our bodies where cancer does its nasty business. Some of this information is fairly fresh as science goes.

Healthy Cell Membranes Are Smart

Our cell membranes are composed of a layer of certain fats (lipids which repel water) between layers of phosphate molecules (which attract water), and, as we have mentioned before, this multi-layer membrane has many variously shaped protein structures scattered throughout it acting as gates or **receptors** to move substances into and out of cells. Each **receptor** is specific to a particular molecule or ion, such as insulin, estrogen, opiates etc. in the same way that a key is specific to a lock. Earlier we discussed Dr. Candace Pert's landmark discovery of the opiate **receptors** on every cell membrane that proves irrefutably the biological interface of body and mind.

Dr. Bruce Lipton illustrates cell membrane structure using a thick layer of butter sandwiched between two pieces of bread in which pitted olives are scattered throughout the butter in such a way that their "ends" are exposed to the layers. He compares the bread layers to the cell membrane phosphate layers and the butter to the lipid or fat layer. He compares the olives to the protein receptors in cell walls. [1] As a cellular biologist, Dr. Lipton came to realize the cell membrane (not the nucleus as once believed) was the "brain" of the cell determining what enters and leaves the cell essentially acting as a "liquid crystal" with its gates and channels just like a computer's semi-conductor. [2]

Cells also have "effector proteins" within them that affect the life process responses to the stimuli entering the cell through the "receptor proteins". The effectors cannot respond if the receptors can't receive essential life sustaining materials like oxygen. Diets including processed (hydrogenated) fats with electrons purposely removed in order to increase shelf life or to mimic the smooth consistency of butter can essentially disable receptors in cell membranes as well as inhibit normal cellular respiration. If cells can't respire or "breathe", they enter the death spiral and, of course, our bodies must follow.

Dr. Johanna Budwig explains this problem throughout her important book, *Flax Oil As a True Aid Against Arthritis, Heart Infarction, Cancer and Other Diseases.* Popular media implies that all fat is the same and "low fat diets" are healthy. In truth some fats (those processed by hydrogenation) are extremely damaging. [3] Others are absolutely essential because our cell walls are largely made up of fats. We will look further at these "good fats" shortly because we can't have "smart" cell membranes unless we know how to build them.

Dr. Garry Gordon, M.D. D.O., in the book, *The Omega 3 Miracle,* says: "How well (cell) membranes perform depends on the quality of their structure . . . The fatty acids in your diet become the fatty acids on your membranes . . . What you eat is what your cells get - no more and no less.[4] He continues, "The foods you consume determine your inflammatory levels.[5] We can conclude that lifestyle which undermines cell membrane health absolutely forces a body cell into abnormal processes that are part of the "disease state" in which cancer often develops.

Tumor Cells Improvise– If We Let Them

". . .The prime cause of cancer is the replacement of respiration of oxygen in normal body cells by a fermentation of sugar." [6] Dr. Otto Warburg said he found fermentation in every cancer cell he examined. The fermentation Warburg references, however, is within a cascade of events that actually begins with whatever "insult" occurs to send the body into a persistent inflammatory mode eventually interrupting normal life processes - first at the cellular level and then at the whole body level. We won't delve into the cascade of events that includes blocked oxidation here, but you can find it expanded in Appendix Five.

Dr. Johanna Budwig explained Warburg's point further saying: "Otto Warburg, in thorough work, determined that all tissue in the living organism, wherever a tumor can be formed, is characterized by the fact that it can no longer absorb oxygen." [7]

Here, we need to consider the direct link between cell membrane integrity and the blockage of oxygen that forces the fermentation.

We have noted that, when body cells are struggling against sustained inflammation from reaction to damaging lifestyle, chronic "insult", or other trauma, oxygen delivery to these cells is interrupted forcing them into abnormal "survival mode" which includes anaerobic fermentation rather than normal "respiration". Cells do what they can to stay alive but fermentation cannot support normal healthy life functions indefinitely.

Among the protein receptors we earlier mentioned there are "pump mechanisms" in cell membranes needing oxygen to generate electrical energy for the cell and for the body.

Realizing that getting oxygen to cells was critical to avoid tumor-enhancing fermentation, Dr. Warburg searched for high-energy fatty acids that are essential for cellular energy generation. He tried some saturated fats that didn't work (we now know) because of the electron type and arrangement within the fat molecule.

As quantum physics arose, scientists realized that photon rich unsaturated fatty acids provide the energy for transporting oxygen in and out of cells. **Un**saturated fats let their electrons easily jump back and forth between molecules thereby generating energy not unlike a solar panel works.

All life processes ultimately depend on sunlight because sunlight transforms into photons, electrons, and particles called "pi-electrons". These solar particles (photons) come to us in plant-based food through the process of photosynthesis (a chemical process using chlorophyll and sunlight). Photons are to light what electrons are to matter and Einstein showed that photons can be energy waves and particles at the same time.

Dr. Johanna Budwig followed Warburg's work concluding: **"The electrons in our food serve as the resonance system for the sun's energy. The electrons in our food are truly the element of life."** [8]

Budwig realized cell membranes were basically "tarred over" by lifeless dietary saturated fats and especially by hydrogenated margarines and nut butters. **Impaired cell membranes exacerbate "blocked oxygen" and other issues.**

"Energy generation" depends on electrons absorbing photons through vibration (resonance), which is the basic energy of everything. Einstein showed that energy and matter are never actually destroyed but merely change form. Therefore, everything is some type of vibration, which means every particle in the universe is connected to every other particle through vibration as we've referenced earlier with Bruce Lipton's and David Van Koevering's comments. Just contemplate being in "resonance" with Holy Spirit within this amazing universe. This intimate relationship is God's expressed intent throughout His Word and in His "Word Made Flesh". (See John 16:13, Romans 8:11, John 1:14.)

When electrons absorb photons they increase their energy levels. Electrons can also give off photons, which involves a great deal of energy and is part of every change of substance in the universe. Dr. Warburg looked for an edible source of this dynamic exchange and didn't find it. Later, Dr. Budwig found that "essential fatty acids" or EFA's plentiful in flax seed possess the particular electron arrangement and type of chemical bonds to transfer tremendous amounts of energy.

We now know that the electron configuration found in flax seeds, walnuts, carotene, and other plant substances provide the energy for oxidation to overcome the anaerobic fermentation in cancerous cells. Wild coldwater fish that ingest plankton also provide EFA's.

Now, we have a deeper realization of the critical importance of "blocked oxygenation" in the cascade of events resulting in the "disease state" that a sustained inflammatory response initiates. Pain is also a result of blocked oxidation.

These highly unsaturated fats Dr. Budwig used are called "**essential** fatty acids" because they can ONLY come from God manufactured food and NOT from humanly processed food. **I hope you are starting to realize we are designed to eat fresh raw vegetables in which photosynthesis has occurred as a way of "eating sunshine".**

We have photons in every healthy body cell . . . We have light in us. After all, Jesus called us *"the light of the world."* (Matthew 5:14) "According to the computable findings of modern physicists, the quantum biologists, there is no entity in nature, in life, which has a higher concentration of solar electrons than man. It then follows that man has a true rapport with sunlight. Physicists today are recognizing more and more that *"Let there be light!"* at the outset of Creation is becoming physically ever clearer to our minds, as the TRUTH." [9]

Fats? For Health? Absolutely!

To steward "the healthy state", we MUST eat fats every day in roughly a 1:1 ratio of Omega 6 and Omega 3 fatty acids (EFA's) for cell membranes to be healthy. The consensus of my reading, however, says that Americans average about 20:1 (Omega-6 to Omega-3) which is highly inflammatory and pushes us into the "diseased state". Omega 6 fatty acids are inflammatory in that they support the normal immune actions of inflammation such as wound healing, but **we are in trouble when we are out of balance toward the inflammatory side.** Omega 3 fatty acids are anti-inflammatory and we are about to discuss ways to positively impact cells in the "diseased state" via the "Budwig Protocol" using omega-3's. At least my own experience with the "Budwig Protocol" has been very positive; although, again, you would want to tune into God to learn if it suits your healing needs.

We earlier noted that the fat consumption directly leading to very unhealthy cell membranes and inflammation is mainly animal fat, highly processed fats, and certain cooking oils. Many people misunderstand the tricky marketing of "low fat", "fat free", and other food labels thinking we need to totally avoid all fats. Not so! We must know how to get the right balance of fatty acids into our diet. I eat a lot of avocados, walnuts, raw almonds, and various seed foods. Walnuts have some of the same fatty acids as flax seeds and I try to eat a handful of walnuts daily.

One other thing to realize about dietary fat is that about 95% of the Essential Fatty Acids we ingest will be used in their original form and about 5% will be converted to DHA, GLA, and EPA which are specifically important for building certain cell membranes (like brain cells for DHA), but taking supplements of these derivatives gets back into the manufactured chemical world which we are generally better off to avoid. If we get the proper Omega 6 and Omega 3 EFA's balanced in our diet, we will have enough to derive all the important fatty acids naturally. Fish oil? I don't take it for many well publicized reasons. I eat a little **wild caught** salmon when available. Keep in mind the "fatty acid balance" is really about helping minimize the chronic inflammation, which we see in the "disease state".

Dr. Richard Firshein, D.O., in *The Nutraceutical Revolution,* writes, "Inflammation is a chemical fire (in our body). [10] He goes on to describe the natural temporary "fever" or "swollen area" meant to facilitate healing and contrasts it with the "fire that won't burn out" kind of inflammation "gone awry" that begs for anti-inflammatory Omega-3 fatty acids to extinguish. Firshein says there have been thousands of scientific studies done on these EFA's in the last decade. "These days, the dietary availability of omega-3 fatty acids in America is only 20 percent of what it was a century ago. "With this plunge, use of corn oils and other high Omega-6 fats has risen. We have also seen increase in "farm raised" or "Atlantic salmon" which is essentially "feed lot" fish fed food pellets (with high corn content) **instead of their natural photon rich plankton**, and, because of unnatural crowded environment, they get antibiotics we don't want in our food. Thus, farm raised salmon is a source of omega-6 while wild caught is a source of omega 3. [11]

I encourage you to "customize" your fat intake as you do every part of your healthy lifestyle. Dialogue with the Lord. No detail is too small to bring to Him.

Here's a Way to 'Eat Sunshine' So Cells Can Breathe

Very early in my change to an "anti-cancer lifestyle" I discovered the already mentioned "Budwig Protocol" in Bill Henderson's *Cancer Free* book.[12] I found this "protocol" helpful and easy for getting essential fatty acids long before I understood why I needed them. For the first two plus years after my "strike two surgery", I also kept my diet strictly vegan except for this protocol. I still limit dairy in my diet to these sulfur rich proteins I mix with flax oil and a bit of organic cheese.

Dr. Budwig, as both researcher and a practitioner, discovered that the essential fatty acids in flax oil combine well chemically with high sulfur proteins making it ideal for unblocking cellular respiration. Electron rich flax seed oil became her choice for the necessary fatty acids. Being German, she used a cottage cheese called "quark".

Flax oil's useful structure also makes it somewhat fragile so that it must be kept cold and in a light barrier container or it will become rancid more quickly than other oils. Flax oil cannot be heated. Olive oil, avocado oil, and coconut oil have their uses in "healthy cooking" but they are not as highly unsaturated as flax oil which means they won't readily combine with protein and function as the energy source we need at the cellular level. Cottage cheese, yogurt, and kefir can be substituted for Budwig's "quark" (organic).

People ask me if flax seeds in a salad or smoothie are as effective as the oil/protein mix. If the seeds are fresh and you use them immediately after they are ground (in a coffee bean grinder), they are helpful and sometimes I do eat them that way; however, this does not expedite the same biochemical function as the "oil-protein" combination which has innumerable testimonies to its success and I am one of them. The seeds, like the oil, must be kept in the cold and dark.

You can find Dr. Budwig's own specific program and recipe recommendations in her books listed in Appendix Two but I've included a few for you below. And you will find some banter about her "protocol" online including a few detractors - mostly orthodox medical folks who mean well but can't shuck their indoctrination that food is basically inert. Further, much of the literature on Budwig's work was originally published in German and only translated to English in the 1990's.

Budwig Smoothie:

I use a blender and put in about a cup of organic kefir (yogurt milk), about 1.5 tablespoons of Barleans organic cold pressed Flax Oil, frozen organic blueberries, strawberries, pineapple, peach slice, raspberries (you choose). Frozen berries work best and a drop of Stevia sweetens. I don't labor over the measuring.

Budwig Yogurt Treat:

I make yogurt but you can buy organic plain. Quantities are approximate. I use about 1/2 cup of yogurt, 1 tablespoons of the flax oil and a little Stevia, fresh organic berries and walnut pieces. Remember my physician friend's advice to "eat lots of blueberries". She was correct . . . and raspberries and strawberries. Organic is worth the price.

Budwig Cottage Cheese Salad Dressing:

I make a salad dressing with organic low fat cottage cheese, flax oil, garlic, and dried herbs (Braggs Sprinkles are good). I just mash the cottage cheese and a generous squirt of flax oil in and mix with a fork. You can see the oil become soluble and add a bit more if you want. Let it set while you make your salad. Put a variety of fresh raw organic vegetables in your salad . . . the more colorful the better. I highly recommend a nice big raw vegetable salad for at least one meal per day. The Hallelujah Acres website, www.hacres.com provides many wonderful salad recipes for health and variety.

I use Barleans Flax Oil available online and, possibly, in local whole food sections of groceries. I actually have a standing order for this oil to be shipped monthly via www.amazon.com. I keep one or two in the freezer as well. I consider it liquid sunshine. I also use Barleans organic coconut oil sparingly as "butter".

Our Whole Body "Membrane" Needs Sunlight Too.

Much is written in "cancer literature" lately about how important Vitamin D is in preventing cancer. Science is quite solid that it is only exposure to sunlight on our skin that enables us to make actual vitamin D. I understand that "vitamin D2 and D3" are sold in bottles and added to food; however, it is hardly a substitute for sunlight's yield. Such chemicals made in a lab to "mimic" part of real vitamin D are actually steroidal hormones. I once started to supplement with "vitamin D3" but never had peace with it. Dr. Steve Blake says in *Vitamins and Minerals Demystified:* "Vitamin D is necessary in the diet only for people who get too little sun to make their own." [13] "Sunlight exposure provides most people with their entire vitamin D requirement. Older people have a slightly diminished capacity to synthesize vitamin D, so they need a little more sun. Also, many older people use sunscreen and wear protective clothing, which limits vitamin D production. Sunscreen with SFP factor of 8 curtails production of vitamin D by 95 percent." [14] Blake discusses skin color and home latitudes as variables. Vitamin D may be supplemented naturally in diet by eating wild caught salmon, sardines, mackerel, herring, tuna, or taking cod liver oil.

Synthetic vitamins are not the same as God made substances and, like all man-made chemicals, don't resonate per our "design". The natural vitamin synthesis process adjusts in many complex ways to our environment and individual needs. Nothing from a bottle can naturally respond in such a way. Look at it this way: I'm an artist and, since "waking up" from cancer, natural colors have appeared far more brilliant to me. My paintings have been more colorful than ever in my life (see some on my blogs), but I still cannot match on paper or canvas, the colors in nature. Color is vibrating light. No artist can match exactly the colors in Creation. The vibrations are simply not the same.

God makes the substances with the energy we need and puts them in sunlight and food. There is NO "vitamin enriched processed food or man-made vitamin" that matches God made! Products labeled "natural" may not be what the name implies.

Fear of Sunshine - An Enemy Counterfeit?

But unto you who revere and worshipfully fear (respect) My name shall the Sun of Righteousness arise with healing in His wings and His beams, and you shall go forth and gambol like calves [released] from the stall and leap for joy. (Malachi 4:2, AMP)

We require the benefits of solar exposure while fear of sunlight has many folks slathering "sun screen" chemicals on their highly absorbent skin. I've sat in oncology clinic waiting rooms crowded with gray skinned people often discussing how doctors told them to avoid sunlight and raw food. The well-documented reason is that these cancer patients have had their life force almost totally insulted by negative energy through "chemotherapy" or "irradiation" purposely deteriorating their immune systems. Many I've spoken with hate life itself as they are warned by treatment providers to avoid their very life force as though it is their enemy. Dr Johanna Budwig also speaks of this phenomenon saying, "Doctors tell cancer patients that they should avoid the sun; that they can't tolerate it. That is correct." [15] So far I've cited a great deal of "sun phobia" without yet mentioning skin cancer. I will shortly.

First, there is good news from Dr. Budwig who follows her above statement with, "The moment, however, that these patients (cancer patients as well) have been following my oil/protein nutritional advice for two or three days, which means that they have been getting sufficient amounts of the essential fats, they can then tolerate the sun very well. Indeed they emphasize how much their vitality and vigor is stirred and stimulated." She explains that this dramatic improvement results from the very energizing at the cellular level through the restoration of the electron exchange her oil-protein protocol enables. Healthy people can and must enjoy sunlight and its benefits if they approach exposure sensibly moving in and out of shade using common sense and protective clothing.[16]

There is additional good news regarding sunlight and health clearly explained by Shane Ellison, M.S., who says that sunlight enables "a family of chemical cousins" called isomers in our skin to, long term, ward off cancer and other diseases. However synthetic vitamin D chemicals bring about a synthesis that builds up on fatty tissue of the body and leads to calcifications, which cause heart, kidney and other organ issues. [17]

Regarding our "love/fear relationship with sunlight", let's put the fear aside and consider sunlight exposure without the panic, Ellison summarizes: "The "ozone layer panic" is well hyped as increasing UV exposure by 20%, but it is done so without realizing that UV exposure can increase by 5,000% just by traveling from pole to equator or going on a tropical vacation because of the changing angle of the sun's rays. Also ignored is the fact that skin cancer rates are lower among people living in areas of strong UV exposure." [18] My own opinion is that sometimes fear is cultivated to further ideological agendas or create demand for products. We know that fear is a powerful counterfeit ploy. No wonder the most frequent command in the Bible is "don't be afraid".

Nevertheless, Ellison points out that, "We have lived under the same sun for millennia. The rate of skin cancer has just begun to grow rapidly and it has been increasing every year . . . .While skin cancer has become a growing threat, the sun has remained unchanged in its actions. Logic dictates that the increased incidence of skin cancer cannot solely be explained by exposure to the sun." [19] Ellison cites a study in the *American Journal of Public Health* when he concludes, "The more sun block you use, the greater your risk of cancer." [120] Since its widespread use from 1950 to 1990, deaths from skin cancer have doubled in women and tripled among men!" [21] Personally, I quit using sunscreen when I entered the "anti-cancer lifestyle" which included Dr. Budwig's flax oil/protein protocol. If I need to be in the sun for more than an hour at a time, I use a totally natural non-toxic product from www.supersalve.com or www.uvnatural.com and wear protective clothing and move in and out of shade.

We MUST Honor Our Largest Organ

Just as our cell membranes are "on the front line" of our inner environment, our largest organ (skin) is on the front line of our outer environment. Our skin absorbs what we rub on it, pour on it, wash over it . . . you get the point. However, we don't think a great deal about our skin's function. We just want it to be pretty and not hurt. We really should think of our skin as "another mouth" regarding toxin intake. Certainly medical science is aware of the skin's absorbing mechanisms because it now uses skin patches for delivery of many kinds of pharmaceuticals.

We've already considered the essential work our skin does absorbing solar electrons and photons and producing vitamin D. Regarding toxicity of chemical sunscreens, I refer you to a well-presented report on the chemicals in sunscreen and encourage you to consider our need for sunlight exposure on our skin and the risks of chemical sun blockers. I encourage you to make your own informed decisions. Our skin provides several square feet of absorbent surface; therefore, what we slather and spray on it is significant. Environmental Working Group link http://www.ewg.org/2013sunscreen/the-trouble-with-sunscreen-chemicals/ provides a good chart of sunscreen chemicals.

Considering care of our skin, there is yet another benefit of Dr. Johanna Budwig's research. She actually compounded what she termed "ELDI (Electron Differentiation) Oils" mixing 75% flax oil with 25% wheat germ oil. She applied this mixture to the skin of some of her patients - particularly late stage cancer patients. She sometimes also used flax oil enemas for those patients. All of Dr. Budwig's flax oil treatment (including nutrition), she writes, brought dramatic healing to her patients so that they could benefit from sunlight exposure.[22]

Turn Back "Stealth Assaults"

Environmental toxins also include many substances absorbed through our skin from household products.

Some dangerous chemicals found in cleaning products include (not a complete list):

Benzene, a solvent and contaminant linked to cancer and male reproductive issues.

Chloroform, a gas that causes cancer and developmental toxicity (children's lungs)

Formaldehyde, a poison with a cumulative effect

If, like me, you hate having to remember a bunch of stuff to avoid, I suggest you consider a positive approach and get rid of all the nasty chemical products in your house and just use simple cleaning substances like:

- ❖ Goat milk soap (on skin)
- ❖ Organic castile soap for everything from bathing to washing the car.
- ❖ Hand soap can also be goat milk, castile or other natural soap
- ❖ Natural fluoride free toothpaste.
- ❖ Simple shampoo and face cleaner base without coloring, fragrances, etc.
- ❖ Simple laundry soap or you can make your own using online recipes
- ❖ White vinegar for mopping floors and windows and many other interior surfaces like countertops.
- ❖ Baking soda which can be made into a paste with water and a little all natural soap and used for scrubbing bathroom fixtures and tile grout.

Fear based advertising has led us into a long season of choosing products to "kill all those nasty germs in our environment that spread disease". A full discussion of this issue is beyond the scope of this book; however, we MUST realize that assumptions we make from a barrage of media propagated fear can be very harmful to our health because it motivates us to purchase and use toxic products that may be more of a danger than the highly touted "germs". We all learned of Louis Pasteur's "theories and discoveries" in school and "modern medicine" is built on Pasteur's "germ theory". Few if any of us were taught about Claude Bernard and Antoine BeChamp's important discoveries and theories.

Pasteur said that the human body was internally pristine without any potentially degrading organisms unless these invaded from the environment. He made no distinction regarding the condition of the body in warding off the invasion so he never explained why everyone exposed to every germ did not get sick. Bernard, BeChamp and Robert Virchow (father of medical pathology) all disagreed with Pasteur and insisted that the condition of the "inner terrain" of a body determined the success of invading organisms. Many historians report that Pasteur, on his death-bed admitted, "Claude Bernard was right. The microbe is nothing. The terrain is everything." Not only did Bernard, BeChamp and Virchow provide sound science as a basis for their theory, they and others have shown that human blood, in fact, contains particles that react to the condition of the "inner terrain" and, of course, when the terrain dies, they work to return it to the dust from whence it came. Several interesting books on this subject are listed in Appendix Two.

I'm not launching a debate on "germ theory", but I do encourage letting go of "germ fear" realizing that we can live a life style that sustains a level of health making our bodies very unlikely hosts for disease regardless of the microbes in the outer environment. We have fearfully and wonderfully made immune systems and many built in defenses. The best defense is health. Several times I have quoted Henry W. Wright saying, "a healthy cell will never become cancerous." [23] In fact, a healthy cell in a healthy terrain is well defended against any disease. We want a clean body and a clean home without moving in fear to wage a war on microorganisms that have little chance to successfully invade a truly healthy body. A swamp can't ward off mosquitos, and a compromised "inner terrain" can't ward off disease germs. This entire book is about sustaining a healthy "inner terrain". Non-toxic cleanliness is part of that endeavor.

Let's Consider Three Often Overlooked Toxin Issues

Pesticides are a particular concern in our food and water. Of course we must avoid toxins where possible, but we have no idea what the wind and aquifer carry through our environment. I take milk thistle every day for liver protection because that organ is on the front line against toxins. Shane Ellison writes, in his book *Over the Counter Natural Cures,* "As a toxicity remedy, milk thistle works in three distinct ways to preserve our health. Once ingested, the active ingredients bind to the squishy membrane of our liver cells to form a protective "shield". This keeps foreign molecules out and essential nutrients in. Milk thistle also protects us from oxygen shock, making it a potent antioxidant. As a natural detoxification cure, it can also serve as a "biological janitor" to clean up foreign molecules. Through a process known technically as conjugation, milk thistle attaches to foreign molecules and carries them out of the body, keeping the liver free from the accumulation of toxic threats. This natural detox cure can be found inexpensively on any grocery store shelf." [24] Thank God for milk thistle!

There are things we use every day like cell phones and other electromagnetic devices and the air around us is filled with energy waves of many shapes and frequencies. Our bodies are very much electrical at the cellular level. We really do not accurately grasp the potential danger of electromagnetic fields; however, we can be reasonably judicious about use of electronics. Should we fear what is in our atmosphere? NO! There is great positive power available in our atmosphere and that is where the focus must be - music, laughter, color, nature, good conversation - there is no end to the good. However, there are few if any good reasons any human being should walk around exposing the "windows of our soul" to a digital screen or holding a potent electromagnetic device near their head or in a pocket near a vital organ. How such habits can be linked to cancer is unclear but other potential damage, to me, seems a "no brainer" starting with a fact cancer teaches well - we can only spend time once and hugging an electromagnetic device is a choice we make. I personally minimize use of the microwave oven as well as other devices.

There is a high statistical link between the incidence of root canals in people experiencing cancer. Bill Henderson has written about this issue. [25] Dr. Andrew Weil, M.D. has also commented about the connection. [26]

Another dental toxin issue is mercury amalgam fillings, which are said to constantly emit various levels of toxic mercury gases. I have had considerable dental work including three root canals that I had checked by a biological dentist to make certain there is not trapped inflammation in my gums. I have also had all mercury fillings either replaced or capped since my "strike two" surgery. I believe this issue is important and would urge you to have your mouth checked out and pray for guidance in making decisions. Screen your dentist to make certain they handle mercury removal properly so you are not inhaling fumes in the removal or capping process.

Detoxification Mechanisms Considered

Throughout the book, we've examined how the considerable fluid in our bodies can become like a "dirty aquarium" or "swampy terrain" in which our body cells struggle to function. We have discussed key and critical ways we can actively and deliberately capitalize on our built in detoxification mechanism- our lymphatic system.

Skillful massage by a trained lymphatic masseuse can be as helpful to lymph movement in skin and muscle tissue as some of the other mechanisms we've discussed are to deeper tissue. With the addition of good music and essential oil aromatherapy, considerable healing benefits ensue.

As I searched resources to instigate my own healing, I waded through a plethora of books that espoused various "detoxification protocols"- many of them requiring the purchase of special products. These "protocols" vary from coffee enemas to colonic irrigation by practitioners using machines. You will need to read about these for yourself. I was not compelled to pursue any of them. I had been cleaned out for digestive tract surgery, and I had bled out requiring my entire blood volume to be replaced by transfusion. God and I agreed that I was not a candidate for any contrived detoxification, except to adopt a lifestyle that would naturally avoid toxins. My body responded by moving through further detoxification quite naturally as I changed my diet and lifestyle including the "lymphasizing mechanisms" I've discussed and nutritional measures I am sharing in this book.

Please fashion your "lymphasizing program" to fit your individual needs. Again, tune in to God for guidance. My purpose has been to introduce you to various ways to maintain lymphatic health. Besides detoxification, the lymphatic system has other essential functions including transporting certain fatty acid molecules from the digestive system to the circulatory system. We have already discussed how fat is essential for the health of our cell membranes and, thereby, the generation of energy. Consequently, the health of our lymphatic system is far more important than most people realize.

Throughout this book, my goal has been to bring you to an understanding that we are designed and empowered by our loving Creator to live in health, peace and joy. We are allowed to choose whether or not our bodies become hospitable to disease - even cancer. The great doctor Albert Schweitzer expressed deep insight into the principle I share by saying, "disease tends to leave me rather rapidly because it finds so little hospitality inside my body." [27] I am alive today because I believed I could make my body inhospitable to cancer. Praise God because, without the revelation of His promises in His Word, I would have had no "standard of universal law" to measure my choices against.

ten

Thirst No More

Remember when I talked about the amazing impact words have upon water? Water we take in has an amazing impact on us as well. Our bodies are largely water. The "healthy state" implies that we must keep the water content of our bodies properly distributed. **Hydration is the single most important element of good health because it facilitates all normal body functions.**

In all my research, one of the most fascinating resources was Dr. F. Batmanghelidg, M.D.'s, *Water for Health, for Healing, for Life*. The tag line in the title is *"You're Not Sick, You're THIRSTY!"* Dr. "Batman" (his chosen nickname) spent his incarceration as an Iranian prisoner of war treating fellow inmates for stress related diseases. He kept careful records of his work so he could share his conclusions. The "take away" points of this book in our context include:

1. "Dry mouth is not the only sign of dehydration."[1] Don't wait until you are thirsty to drink water. "It is now crystal clear that the human body has many different ways of showing its water needs." [2] I list other signs of thirst later.

2. Water is not only "life sustaining" but also "life giving" in its nature. [3] Water is not inert as Dr. Emoto's crystals reveal; rather it holds within it far more cosmic truth than we have realized even though Scripture is rich with lessons regarding "living water"– lessons

often interpreted too figuratively. Water constantly transports life-giving elements to every cell and transports life threatening toxins from every cell. We have seen in Emoto's crystals, that it is somehow part of our soul as well as body.

3. People are deceived "thinking that tea, coffee, alcohol, and manufactured beverages can substitute for the pure natural water needs of the body."[4] "Dr. Batman" says this assumption is "an elementary mistake, particularly in a body that is stressed. It is true that these beverages contain water, but most also contain dehydrating substances such as caffeine . . . "when you drink coffee, tea, or even a beer, your body gets rid of more water than is contained in the drink." [5] **We know that only pure water contains oxygen and hydrogen, which is the only material in a beverage our blood and lymph fluid can use.**

We must keep water "flowing" through our bodies constantly to avoid "stagnation". Doctors Guyton and Hall, in *The Textbook of Medical Physiology, 11th Ed.,* explain, "The kidneys must continually excrete at least some fluid, even in a dehydrated person, to rid the body of excess solutes that are ingested or produced by metabolism. Water is also lost by evaporation from the lungs and the gastrointestinal tract and by evaporation and sweating from the skin. Therefore, there is always a tendency for dehydration, with the resultant increased extracellular fluid sodium concentration." Additionally there is a threshold for drinking at a certain sodium concentration in the extracellular fluid. "Water intake restores extracellular fluid osmolality (movement through membranes) and volume toward normal." [6] Earlier, when we were discussing the various receptors on cell membranes, I mentioned that one of them was a pump requiring oxygen to generate energy. That pump relies on proper sodium concentration in the fluid between cells. "Dr. Batman" adds, **"All living and growing species, humans included, survive as a result of energy generation from water."** [7]

All Drinks are NOT Water

Media is packed with energy booster drinks hyped to overcome that "afternoon slump" capitalizing on the everyone-does-it lifestyle. Even the pink ribbon disease marketing campaign now participates in this health counterfeit. "Dr. Batman", however, can save us some grief and money as he teaches regarding feeling tired without a plausible reason. He says, "**Water is the main source of energy formation in the body**. Even the food that is supposed to be a good source of energy has no value to the body until it is hydrolyzed by water and energized in the process."[8] Until recently, car batteries required monitoring of their water level to keep the current flowing. Now they are "closed cell" so water is not lost. We saw in previous chapters that electrical energy generation at the cellular level is an essential life process. Guess what, we still have to monitor and maintain our body's "battery" water level. Pure water or liquid "Foo Foo Dust" for energy boost? No contest!

"Dr. Batman" also gives other body thirst signs such as unreasonable irritability, dejection, feelings of inadequacy, autoimmune maladies and depression. He also discusses short attention span, quick temper, flushing, shortness of breath, cravings for manufactured beverages and alcohol, feeling "heavy headed" and disturbed sleep as "body thirst" signals.[9] Many of these things are linked to acid/alkaline imbalance from dehydration triggered situations in the body such as loss of amino acids (proteins) and insufficient absorption or loss of certain minerals and the absolute need for essential vitamins and **fatty acids**." [10] **Nearly every book or study I've read points out that cancer thrives in an acidic body environment and even perpetuates that condition as it progresses.** Drs. Batman and Budwig compliment each other well.

How Do We Get the Water We Need?

We need to drink about half our "body weight" in water per day in ounces. If I weigh 130 pounds, I need to drink a minimum 65 ounces (2+ quarts) of water per day and more if exercising because the average loss is 3.5

quarts per day. Water in vegetable juice counts. Water in fruit juice is so full of sugar without the buffering fiber of whole fruit it's not recommended. Fresh fruits and vegetables have good water content and that's a bonus for me because I eat a lot of them but don't count them in my water intake goal. **It is best to avoid foods that make us thirsty.**

Bottled water? Some people find bottled natural spring water acceptable. I don't like to drink anything that has spent a lot of time in plastic containers, and particularly if it may have spent time in hot temperatures such as a truck or rail car. I use a stainless steel portable water bottle and carry my filtered water with me. Regarding purity of bottled water, Dr. Andrew Weil, M.D. cited a study done at the University of Iowa of 10 brands of bottled water showed "cancer causing contaminants in the store brands of several large retail chains at levels the same as those routinely found in tap water." [11]

Tap Water? Fluoride, Chlorine, discarded pharmaceutical residue, agricultural run off, and a few other issues exist in public water supplies. Refrigerator filter quality varies and I've seen none that filter out all the total dissolved solids in tap water. I'm not going to launch a technical discussion of how these toxins get into the water. I note that that the "city water" in my community comes from a brand new treatment plant and my digital meter regularly reads 135 to 225 total dissolved solids per the national standard unit of measure. This amount it acceptable by government standards - actually about average. I'd rather have water with a zero reading.

What do I do? In the first several years post cancer, I drank only distilled water processed from a countertop distiller. Yes, rock minerals are distilled out of water, but only plants can use those. We must get our minerals from those plants. A distiller uses more energy and time than I wanted to invest.

Now, I use a Zero Water Filter purchased online for about $50 which uses zero electricity to bring my water to zero "total dissolved solids" content. This filter and countertop reservoir comes with a digital meter to alert me to replace filter at a reading of 0.06. I spend about $50 per year on filter cartridges. It is a neat process.

Some people have whole house water filters or distillers. It is a personal choice and costs vary. I have recently started using a hand-held showerhead filter knowing our skin so readily absorbs what is in our bath water and I like to relax in the bath.

The next section on juicing fits closely with our discussion of drinking plenty of pure water because, while some may wonder about giving up bulky cellulose fiber in vegetables through juicing, we need to realize the benefit in picking up water "filtered and electrically balanced by nature itself"– particularly from organic vegetables. Drinking fresh vegetable juice is like an "express delivery" of concentrated nutrients to every cell without taxing the digestive system in the process.

Notes:

Section IV

The Power of Food to Restore Health

"Let food be thy medicine and medicine be thy food!"
  Hippocrates (460-377 b.c.)

eleven

Embracing the Power of Food

One of the "side effects" to entering the world of good nutrition was a pleasant surprise to me. There I was "in the valley of the shadow of death" and God *"prepared a table before me in the presence of my enemies, anointed my head with oil, and filled my cup to overflowing"* (Psalms 23). The coolest part of all was that what He put on this table made me feel INCREDIBLE right away and it still does. What amazing energy a healthy lifestyle provides! Just ask my three active grandchildren who beats them back up the sleigh riding hill. At my Real Health Hope Seminars people have asked, "Am I going to have to keep this 'diet' up the rest of my life?"

My answer is quick and sure: "It is not a diet and it makes you feel so incredible, you would never think of jumping off this wagon." It is not bondage and you won't turn into a turnip if you eat one cookie, but you absolutely will become addicted to feeling amazingly energetic and light so that, if you occasionally hop off the wagon, you will run to catch up and get back on.

I promise! NOTHING feels better than health because you find yourself as one of "those" Isaiah 40:31 describes: ... *but **those** who hope in the LORD will renew their strength. They will soar on wings like eagles; they will run and not grow weary, they will walk and not faint.* (NIV)

After my "strike two surgery", I was trying to get my healing program underway and struggled to find information. I remain grateful for Bill

Henderson's *Cancer Free: Your Guide to Gentle, Non-Toxic Healing.* Bill doesn't deal with spiritual aspects, but he introduced me to the Budwig protocol, Beta Glucan, Barley Power, and *The China Study.* I appreciate this "Anti-Cancer Crusader's" relentless work. If you want a synopsis of a great many alternative cancer treatments, Bill's book includes a bunch of them as does his eNewsletter. I was not looking for a "treatment", however. I wanted my body sustainably inhospitable to cancer. Bill recommends a particular daily vitamin/mineral product that I took for about a year; then I read Dr. Norman Walker's books on juicing and decided I wanted to get all my vitamins and nutrients from fresh vegetables. Walker used juicing to overcome severe health problems as a young man and lived a vibrant and active life to age 100+. I like to have long-term personal testimonies for the protocols I use.

Besides Walker's books, I read Dr. George Malkmus' book, *The Hallelujah Diet,* about Malkmus' personal story of using juicing and a vegetable diet to overcome colon cancer many decades ago shortly after losing his mother who chose "orthodox cancer treatment". Rev. Malkmus is now a vibrant 80+ year old. His website, www.hacres.com, has many good resources including recipes.

Juicing:

I am going to share my juicing program but you can adapt your own. I prefer to make a pint of fresh juice every morning (10 minutes), but sometimes I make juice for about five days at a time and refrigerate it in pint size glass canning jars with plastic lids. I make the juice and mix it in a glass container with a spout and then I fill the jars to the brim so that little if any air can be present. I have two juicers. One is a Hamilton Beach centrifugal juicer that is pretty quick to use. It does an adequate job but does mix some air into the juice that may affect its "nutritional storage life". I also have is a Solo Star II with a ceramic auger. It is a bit slower but quieter and it crushes leafy vegetables as well as others and gets all the juice out. The Solo Star II is somewhat easier to clean than the centrifugal juicer and it has a pasta "nozzle" as well as a blank to use making a neat "soft serve dessert" made from freshly frozen bananas and berries. Later I discuss sprouted grain flour useful in making fresh pastas.

Choice of juice vegetables is personal and God certainly will help you know what your body needs. It's fun to experiment with mixtures. I use carrots, celery, cucumbers, peppers, beets, kale, etc depending on what "I have a sense for at the market". I keep carrot and beet amounts below others because of glycemic index (sugar) in these. I don't add fruit as some do to make the juice more cleansing. Immediately before drinking, I add one scoop of a good "greens powder" like BarleyMax from Hallelujah Acres. They sell a neat shaker cup I mix it in and drink it from.

My preparation of the vegetables is simple. I wash (sometimes soak them in a sink filled with ice water and a little white vinegar for an hour to make washing large amounts easier), trim, peel as necessary and feed into juicer. My entire process including prep, juicing and clean up for 5 pints is about an hour. Once you get your routine down, it is quick and easy. Just turn on the music and enjoy it.

I drink a pint of this juice first thing every morning. I wouldn't miss my juice because it makes me feel so good. One pint of juice yields the nutrients from a whole cucumber, three carrots, and a small bunch of celery in my usual blend. I compost the residual fiber.

Traveling, I carry a small cooler with a few jars of my juice. I sometimes use the BarleyMax powder in pure water as a temporary substitute. Shake don't stir.

Smoothies:

Smoothies are a quick, easy salad meal that can be safely "eaten" on the way to wherever you're going. Smoothies expedite "delivery of the best groceries to our cells", and my own experience is that they sustain an amazing energy that lasts for hours if I continue to drink good water. I often have a smoothie for lunch and never think about food again until dinner. It is good to chew something along with drinking a smoothie to get full digestive processes flowing. I like nut crackers or raw almonds.

There are tons of smoothie recipes in books and online, but I like to make up my own. By now you may realize I keep my diet and health maintenance simple - resting in God all the way rather than trying to follow a lot of "sure fire protocols" or "must do" remedies. The pursuit of health (or muscles, money or whatever) can become an idol itself. What matters is pursuing the Healer and He will BE our health. I pause to focus on our Creator/Healer here in the middle of our discussions of food, exercise, and lifestyle matters because our eating, drinking, exercising, etc. mean nothing if we are not doing these things with the constant awareness that they are components of stewarding God given health.

I have mentioned that God may "turn your attention" toward a food your body needs. I have been strongly compelled to add certain foods to my diet at particular times. One is avocados. I never ate them previously but now they are a staple.

Let's remember, as Exodus 15:26 teaches that God said, *"For I am the Lord who heals you."* Marilyn Hickey, one of my favorite "cut to the chase" teachers points out, "God literally said, *'I am your health'*!"[1]

Returning to smoothies, my all time favorite is one a fellow pancreatic cancer survivor shared with me online.

Kelly's Smoothie:

- ❖ Handful of fresh spinach washed (organic or home grown)
- ❖ One avocado (just cut in half and scoop it out with a spoon discarding pit and skin)
- ❖ Handful of berries– strawberry, raspberry, blueberry in any combo you like (fresh or frozen)
- ❖ Two or three pieces of peach or mango (fresh or frozen)
- ❖ Fill in with coconut milk or water (water works best I think)

I sometimes add a few fresh ground flax seeds. Blend and enjoy! The colors of the ingredients (red and green) may make the smoothie a bit "beige" but you won't mind because it tastes incredible and, again, you feel uplifted immediately. Grab a handful of raw nuts or nutcrackers and make a meal of it.

VITAMIN C - We Need the Real Thing

If you want to read a lot of conflicting information, you can find much about vitamin C and cancer. Let's not wade in muddied scientific waters.

When I went to a good naturopathic doctor several years ago, she helped me understand the difference between vitamin supplements and vitamins in food– particularly C. I decided I wanted the real thing. So I got an inexpensive citrus juicer and keep a quart glass jar with a plastic lid of fresh squeezed organic lemon juice in my refrigerator at all times. I enjoy a bit in some of my herbal and green teas and I like fresh lemonade made with Stevia and filtered water. I drink about 4 ounces of lemon juice daily and I know I get a good ration of real C which is a potent antioxidant that can neutralize a free radical without becoming one itself.

Vitamin C is also important in forming healthy collagen connective tissue (critical for skin elasticity). "Vitamin C can also protect many indispensable molecules in the body, such as proteins, fats, carbohydrates, and nucleic acids (DNA and RNA) from oxidative damage which is one way it can help reduce the risk of cancer." [2]

For those of you wondering if lemon juice isn't "too acidic", its metabolized "ash" is not acidic. Some warn against drinking lemonade with meals. I drink it when I want to.

Alkalinity Help is Here

To help sustain a consistently alkaline "cell terrain" within the scope of my anti-cancer lifestyle, I take Barley Power tablets from Green Supreme at www.greensupreme.net who also sells litmus paper which I use every single morning checking either first urine or saliva for pH reading to keep track of trends over time. I don't panic if an isolated day tests a bit acidic. I take seven "Barley Power" tablets about thirty minutes before each meal. They are "just plain good food". If I forget, I just take them with the meal.

There is much written about the importance of maintaining our body's natural slightly alkaline status. In Appendix Two, I list books indexing foods promoting acidity or alkalinity. Dr. Johanna Budwig speaks to the link between acid/alkaline body chemistry and essential fatty acids we discussed earlier saying: "The acid/alkaline balance will only be restored if highly unsaturated fats are restored as the natural basis in the vital function in blood and in the lymph of the person through a natural supply of natural seed oils with highly unsaturated fats. All other functions are important and remain important, but the base disturbance must be resolved." [3]

Our blood must remain just slightly alkaline or we die. The Standard American Diet generally tilts our biochemistry decidedly toward acidity especially with the Omega-6 fatty acid surplus so prevalent. An anti-inflammatory diet rich in fresh vegetables, (and fruits to a lesser extent), with extremely minimal meat and dairy tilts us back toward alkalinity. The point is that cancer thrives in acidity; however we don't want to force an extreme condition either way. Balance is key.

While our diet impacts our bodily pH level (acidity), we have already discussed at length other factors that lead to the acidic "disease state" in our bodies. Acidity can be cause or effect because cells forced into fermentation produce lactic acid. Diet alone may not maintain a slightly alkaline biochemistry. We have already discussed at length other toxins that lead to the chronic inflammatory and the acidic conditions cancer loves. Our bodies will strive to survive and, if necessary, rob our bones of calcium to offset acidity. In my seminars, people often ask about supplementing with calcium when they learn I eat little dairy. Fresh vegetables (and fruits) have considerable natural calcium in them. I've never taken or needed calcium supplements and my bone density is good. You may need to monitor yours but, again, a natural food source is safer than manufactured calcium sources.

Stealth Sugar

In my seminars, people often groan audibly when I call sugar "cancer fertilizer". However, I assure them they can't beat me in the intensity of my own "sugar habit" that I'm now delivered from. I'm not kidding when I say "delivered from" because I agree with those who see sugar addiction is a diabolic ploy - the result of a non-personal commercialized food supply many believe is intentionally chocked full of addicting sugar disguised by "more marketable names" like "cane syrup", "milk sugars", "high fructose corn syrup", "raw sugar", etc.

Are some food manufacturers intentionally assuring consumers "can't eat just one"? Much is written on this subject, but I choose to forego the "fear campaigns" and just make healthy choices avoiding processed foods. I have a life to live and I know what to eat that allows me to do so. I don't have time to worry about "missing out on some sports drink that looks like window cleaner" or cookies made by elves. The ONE *in me is greater than he that is in the world* (see 1 John 4:4), and I know which foods are "of the world" and which ones are in the form God made them. I promise you that you can't eat harmful food and take "medicine" to overcome the damage. Here are some good "rules of thumb":

- ❖ Avoid anything served to you through your car window.
- ❖ Shop the fresh produce (especially organic) section of the market then go check out
- ❖ Support local farmers' produce markets.
- ❖ Read the labels on packages carefully because sugar is usually added to processed foods labeled as "natural".
- ❖ Remember the enemy is a counterfeiter and, as Eve found out, he does devious food commercials.

Yes, there is fructose sugar in fresh fruit which requires a fairly complicated liver process to digest so we want it only in its natural form buffered with the high fiber built in to fruits rather than juiced to concentrate the sugar. Commercial juices are usually loaded with natural fructose as well as added sugars, artificial colors, and preservatives. I stick to peaches, apples and lots of berries as my main fruit sources.

Highly concentrated corn syrup (HFCS) is lethal over time and it is in nearly every "processed food" from soda pop to processed meat. Other forms of sugar are just as pervasive in packaged food and are equally addictive. Sports drinks are loaded with these sugars as are breads and even "health food" or "breakfast" bars. You will feel wonderful having knocked the sugar monkey off your back. A lot of people deceive themselves trying to "have their cake and eat it too" using artificial sweeteners– especially in soft drinks.

Artificial Sweeteners are a Chemical Issue

The idea that "artificial sweeteners" are healthier than sugar is a lie. Otherwise intelligent people constantly fall for this diabolic marketing ploy. These substances are toxic chemicals. In her book, *Everything You Need to Know to Feel Go(o)d,* brilliant pharmacologist, biochemist and former diet soda drinker, Candace Pert, PhD, writes about the chemical, Aspartame, marketed as NutraSweet, Equal, and Spoonful (in the UK) with great concern for its toxicity. [4]

If you consume foods laced with aspartame, I encourage you to get more information about this chemical which Dr Pert explains, "is a peptide consisting of two amino acids, phenylalanine and aspartic acid, which occur naturally in foods we eat in small quantities. Both of these amino acids are known as excititoxins, which can cause neurons (brain cells) to become overexcited to the point of burnout and death. Monosodium glutamate (MSG) also falls into this category." [5] Dr. Pert walks her reader through the imbalances in neurotransmitter ratios this chemical can set off the impact of which can be "panic symptoms, mood disorders; and for some people, altered seizure thresholds, leading to convulsions." [6]

Dr. Pert goes on to explain in layman's terms how phenylalanine, a third component of aspartame breaks down into methanol which, alone (not in certain foods), is "wood alcohol" the liver breaks down into an even more toxic substance, formaldehyde, long listed as a carcinogen but also used to embalm dead bodies. [7]

Regarding potency factors involved with aspartame as an artificial sweetener Pert explains, "As a pharmacologist, I know that the dosage of a drug is a determining factor for toxicity. The higher the dose, the higher the chance of toxic effect. But another factor, the *potency*, contributes to the dosage. Some drugs are so potent that only small doses are needed, such as the opiate etorphine, which is used in tranquilizer guns to stop a 900 pound charging rhinoceros in its tracks." [8]

Continuing, Dr. Pert explains: "NutraSweet, I found out, isn't very potent, so large quantities are required to bring about its sweet effect. One can of soda contains an amount of aspartame that would fill half the center of my cupped hand. That's an awful lot of methanol and formaldehyde for the body to deal with, . . ." She concludes, "My own review of the literature supports a policy of zero tolerance, regardless of studies claiming to show acceptable levels for daily intake." [9]

I'm compelled to inform you about a movie Dr. Pert references entitled "Sweet Misery" available online. Dr. Pert shares that she personally researched the information in this movie after receiving a copy during a book signing. I think you will find the science and its implications for health and healing astounding. The filmmaker is a young woman who was extremely ill and diagnosed with MS. She did not take ownership of that diagnosis and "acted on instinct" eliminating the two to three diet sodas she drank daily. Dr. Pert relates that this young woman, Cori Brackett, "abruptly began to improve". Cori and her husband convinced her "disease" was a side effect of drinking aspartame laced beverages, made the movie, "Sweet Misery", to warn others. Dr. Pert applauds the purpose and content of this couple's video, and, in her book, adds her own conclusions as I have shared.

Another artificial sweetener, Splenda, is not aspartame. Most people think of it as a safe alternative to sugar. According to Shane Ellison, "the people's chemist", it is not. See my www.realhealthhope.com post entitled "What The People's Chemist Has to Say About Splenda" June 1, 2013.

Ellison says, "Discovered to be 600 times sweeter than sugar, Splenda (sucralose) is a drug that originated as an insecticide but was later used as an artificial sweetener. The molecule contains a historically deadly "organochlorine" or simply: a Really-Nasty Form of Chlorine (RNFOC)." [10]

"Unlike the harmless ionic bond in table salt, The RNFOC in sucralose is a covalent bond." Ellison continues, "When used, the RNFOC yields such poisons as insecticides, pesticides, and herbicides. A RNFOC can invade every nook and cranny of the body. Cell walls and DNA (deoxyribonucleic acid), the genetic map of human life, become potential casualties of war. This may result in weakened immune function, irregular heartbeat, agitation, shortness of breath, skin rashes, headaches, liver and kidney damage, birth defects, and cancer." [11]

Per Ellison, "Hiding its origin, sucralose pushers assert that it is 'made from sugar'. "Sucralose is as close to sugar as glass cleaner is to purified water. France has recently banned such false advertising statements. Burying their head in the sand, the deceit has been ignored by health officials within the USA; sucralose is the most widely used artificial sweetener today." [12]

If you want to overcome or avoid cancer or a number of other common "diseases", I implore you to "get a handle" on sugar and artificial sweeteners. Remember what the prophet Hosea wrote: *"My people perish for lack of knowledge"* (Hosea 4:6). People must "know" the impact of eating either sugar or artificial sweeteners on their health and lifespan.

Sugar IS Cancer Fertilizer

Here's what happens in normal sugar (glucose) metabolism:

- ❖ We take in sugar.
- ❖ Insulin from pancreas hurries to muscle cells carrying glucose (sugar) and nutrients.
- ❖ At cell membrane, insulin is guided to its specific receptors.
- ❖ Normally a chemical bond with phosphorus occurs (phosphorylation) which pulls the sugar (glucose) and nutrients into the cell for use in life processes.

Our miraculous hormonal intelligence shows its power and blood sugar and insulin are controlled by this chemical bonding (phosphorylation) and energy, fat loss, anti-aging hormones flood the body in exactly proper amounts at just the right times. What a Creator we have to cooperate with by keeping our lifestyle within healthy ranges by living in harmony with natural law.

However, if the phosphorylation is messed with because of sugar drenching, we become numb to insulin ("insulin resistant") and:

(a) All subsequent hormonal intelligence quits working giving us belly fat, bad blood, bad moods, inflammation, etc.

(b) Sugar (glucose) and vital nutrients can't get to the aging and insulin resistant cell so these molecules float in the bloodstream and attach to the hemoglobin there.

Patrick Quillin PhD, RD, CNS, writes in *Beating Cancer with Nutrition:* "Elevated sugar in the blood has a number of ways in which it promotes cancer: Rises in blood glucose generate corresponding rises of insulin, which then pushes prostaglandin production toward the immune-suppressing and stickiness-enhancing PGE-2. . . . Potent fatty acids are neutralized when the blood glucose levels are kept high. [My note: Please recall our discussion of electron rich Essential Fatty Acids in the Budwig Protocol.] Cancer cells feed directly on blood glucose, like a fermenting yeast organism. **Elevating blood glucose in a cancer patient is like throwing gasoline on a smoldering fire . . . Elevating blood glucose levels suppresses the immune system.**"[13] (my emphasis) Quillin also discusses the role of sugar (blood glucose) in lowering body pH to acidic and the detrimental impact of acidity in fighting cancer that harkens back to our discussion of Otto Warburg's findings regarding fermentation.

I believe, from my extensive reading, that there is an "expert consensus" on the value of starving cancer cells by cutting sugar out of one's diet. As Dr. Andrew Weil, M.D. says in *Natural Health, Natural Medicine,* "A great many processed foods contain large amounts of sugar to make them taste good. Many condiments such as ketchup, relishes, and pickles are loaded with sugar, as are most soft drinks. The sugar industry likes to tell us that sucrose has only eighteen calories per teaspoon, but most recipes call for *cups* of sugar, and there are a lot of teaspoons in a cup." [14]

Dr. David Servan-Schreiber, M.D./PhD points out that refined sugar, bleached flour, and certain vegetable oils (like corn, safflower, etc) "directly fuel the growth of cancer." [15] He notes as we have before, "The German biologist, Otto Warburg, won the Nobel Prize in medicine for his discovery that the metabolism of malignant tumors is largely dependent on glucose consumption. In fact, the PET scan commonly used to detect cancer simply measures the areas in the body that consume the most glucose. If a particular area stands out because it consumes too much sugar, cancer is very likely the cause." [16] He adds, "There is good reason to believe that the sugar boom contributes to the cancer epidemic." [17]

The above discussion on "sugar as cancer fertilizer" is excerpted from my blog post by that title on: www.realhealthhope.com, October 7, 2010. I hope you will check it out further.

I find the natural herb, Stevia, to be a helpful sweetener. As I've mentioned before, it has zero calories and zero glycemic index so it cannot raise blood sugar levels. A little goes a long way. I have found a number of nice recipes online that use it. Be careful to buy pure Stevia extract and not a mixture with sugar or alcohol.

Sugar is not a Biblical food although honey is and raw organic honey used in moderation may be quite suitable for some people. Unlike the herbal sweetener, Stevia, honey has a glycemic index and must be metabolized as a sugar so moderation makes sense. Dr Andrew Weil says, "As far as carbohydrates are concerned, honey isn't any better or worse for you than sugar, whether or not you have type 2 diabetes. Honey contains fructose, glucose and water plus other sugars as well as trace enzymes, minerals, amino acids and a wide range of B vitamins. The amount of these micronutrients varies depending on where the honey comes from. In general, darker honeys contain more vitamins than lighter ones and also provide more trace minerals such as calcium, magnesium and potassium." [18]

Agave Nectar (from a cactus plant by same name) is also a natural sugar. I haven't used much of it. I occasionally use a tiny bit of raw honey - usually on toast and sprinkled heavily with pure cinnamon a good blood sugar "buffer". Cinnamon is very helpful, but all cinnamon is not equal, you can find a descriptive re-post of a well-researched article by Colleen Story on my blog, www.realhealthhope.com dated October 4, 2013. [19]

What About Salt?

If you curtail your intake of processed and "fast" foods, you will cut an enormous amount of sodium chloride (white table salt) out of your diet. We do need sodium in our bodies but we don't need white table salt. The naturopathic doctor I worked with instructed me to use salt sparingly and to add very little to my food because a diet of mostly fresh vegetables contains enough sodium for health. She advised that any salt I use should be unrefined sea salt and she chose the natural pink "sea salt". She suggested sea vegetable powder and Bragg's organic herb sprinkles to season food. I now enjoy dulse flakes and Bragg's with kelp. The sea vegetables add wonderful nutrients, iodine, and a bit of natural sea salt to food. Dried herbs crumbled up over salads or steamed vegetables are delicious and nutritious. Just approach the "cut down on salt" challenge creatively rather than seeing it as denial. It's all about your attitude and moving toward health rather than away from old habits.

If you want more sodium chloride science, there is a National Institute of Health manuscript online. Just search "Sodium Chloride and Autoimmune Disease" and you will find a Yale led study indicating that sodium chloride is quite inflammatory and the number one source of it in our diets is bread. For bread, I mostly use Ezekiel 4:9 brand (in freezer case because no preservatives added).

Note regarding MSG which I won't discuss here: On my blog www.realhealthhope.com December 1, 2011, there is a nice article about MSG entitled, "Stealth Poison– -By any other name it is still MSG" re-posted from www.Beating-Cancer-Gently.com .

Nutraceuticals are Anti-Cancer Agents in Food

Food is medicine and medicine is food, according to Hippocrates. And God, the Creator of all food, seemed to have this in mind as we see in Genesis 1:29-30:

> *And God said, See, I have given you every plant yielding seed that is on the face of all the land and every tree with seed in its fruit; you shall have them for food.*
> *And to all the animals on the earth and to every bird of the air and to everything that creeps on the ground—to everything in which there is the breath of life—I have given every green plant for food. And it was so. (AMP)*

Hereafter, we will refer to health promoting molecules of nutritional "provisions from Creation" as "Nutraceuticals". Our discussion of nutraceuticals will primarily include an overview of foods that contain naturally occurring molecules which promote several important anti-cancer mechanisms such as apoptosis (cell suicide) and inhibiting angiogenesis (tumors stimulating abnormal blood vessel growth toward themselves) the significance of which we saw earlier.

Nutraceutical foods are best consumed in raw, natural form, but I will sometimes note their supplement forms. I include many of them in my diet and supplement some in order to make absolutely certain I get them consistently. Obviously, several nutraceutical foods are included in the few recipes I've shared but you can get great recipes online at www.hacres.com among other sites.

No list could be fully comprehensive and I will give you additional resources in Appendix Three and Four to enable delving further into this topic. My blog www.realhealthhope.com also has more information regarding dietary supplementation including my sharing what I personally take in an April 2013 post; however, I am NOT recommending or suggesting that you take anything or that you "take what I take". These choices are yours to make as you dialogue with God.

Let your food be your medicine

The book, *Foods to Fight Cancer,* by Dr. Richard Beliveau, PhD and Dr. Denis Gingras, PhD is a magnificent resource for understanding the disease preventing and reversing actions of specific molecules contained within particular foods.[20] The following comparison/contrast of "nutraceuticals" and pharmaceuticals is part of the information within this book as well as in Dr. David Servan-Schreiber's book, *Anti-Cancer: A New Way of Life.*[21]

In Comparison, both Nutraceuticals and Pharmaceuticals have known molecular structures and both have known cellular and molecular targets. However, in contrast:

Nutraceuticals: Molecules Naturally Occurring in Food - Natural

Pharmaceuticals: Created in a laboratory - Synthetic

Nutraceuticals: Selected over the course of history (with survival as motivation).

Pharmaceuticals: Selected in a laboratory (with profit as part of motivation)

Nutraceuticals: NO Side Effects

Pharmaceuticals: PRONOUNCED Side Effects

Nutraceuticals: Synergy or antagonism by design

Pharmaceuticals: Synergy or antagonism due to chance and rarely recognized

No single food or drug is a miracle cure. No single dose or even periodic dose is a miracle cure. It is the consistent and constant intake of a synergistic (beneficially combined) variety of "anti-cancer molecules" that maintain a bright, clean, "healthy state" terrain for cells to thrive and perform their life processes within so that the body is full of vitality. Eating nutraceutically is a lifestyle promoting the "healthy state" that we are looking for.

I repeat, in this vital environment, inflammation and disease state conditions are avoided; apoptosis (suicide of rogue or cancer cells) is facilitated, angiogenesis (the diabolic or "counterfeit" stimulation of blood supply to tumorous tissue) is blocked, and cell walls are clean and active.

Nutraceuticals take advantage of cancer's need to be in a particular environment to thrive by changing that environment chemically and, ultimately, electrically. The discussion of the chemical molecules such as catechins, flavinols, anti-oxidants, etc in nutraceuticals is beyond the scope of this discussion. Be careful about trying to buy these chemical molecules concentrated in pill or capsule form. Extracting the molecules from their food source can render them impotent. Whole food extracts like green tea or turmeric can be helpful to supplement a good diet but not to make up for a poor diet.

Nutraceutical Food is Readily Available

According to Dr. Michail J. Wargovich of M.D. Anderson Hospital, Houston, TX in an article he wrote in "The Cancer Bulletin", "We've found that fruits and vegetables contain a variety of powerful chemicals which interact and bind to chemical carcinogens, rendering them inactive. Some of these chemicals might also interfere with the metabolism of carcinogens rendering them inactive. Some of these chemicals might also interfere with the metabolism of carcinogens in the liver." [22]

Green Tea:

Green tea is rich in polyphenols including catechins, which reduce the growth of new vessels needed for tumor growth & metastases. It is also a powerful antioxidant and detoxifier (activating liver enzymes that eliminate toxins from body, and it facilitates death of cancer cells by apoptosis. Decaf version works just as well. Steep 8-10 minutes covered and drink within an hour of brewing. It is also available as a whole food extract.

Olives and Olive Oil:

Olives are rich in Phenolic anti-oxidants. Black are richer than green especially if not subjected to Spanish style brining. Olive oil should be cold pressed, extra virgin rather than refined and required storage in a dark cool place. 1 to 12 tablespoon per day is usual recommendation. It is an unsaturated fat but not equal to flax oil in EFA provision. Can be used for medium temperature cooking where flax oil cannot.

Ginger:

Ginger root (fresh shredded on a salad or other dish) is powerful anti-inflammatory and anti-oxidant and can also be dried and used as a tea. It is also available separate or combined with garlic in capsule form.

Garlic, Onions, Leeks, Shallots, Chives:

Garlic is one of oldest medicinal foods and known thousands of years b.c. The sulfur compounds of this food family reduce carcinogenic effects of nitrosamines and N-nitroso compounds which are created in grilled meat. They promote apoptosis in cancers manifesting in colon, breast, lung, and prostate as well as leukemia. Studies show high garlic diets have less manifestation of cancer in kidneys and prostate. It also helps regulate blood sugar, reduces insulin secretion and IGF (thus reduces growth of cancer cells). Active molecules of garlic release in crushed clove and assimilated better if combined with olive oil. Available in whole food extract capsule form combined with ginger or by itself. The "odorless" does not include allicin which is a critical ingredient.

Carotenoids:

Lutein, lycopene, phytoene, and canthaxanthin stimulate the growth of immune cells and increase their capacity to attack tumor cells. These include vitamin A and lycopene which have proven capacity to inhibit the growth of several cancer cell lines including brain gliomas.

Vegetables & Fruits rich in Carotenoids include carrots, yams, sweet potatoes, squash, pumpkin, tomatoes, apricots, beets, and all bright colored vegetables. A well researched article by Neev M. Arnell on the benefits of colorful foods is available on www.naturalnews.com (May 20, 2011). [23] This article breaks down foods by color and lists the nutraceutical benefits as well as vegetables within each color category. Obviously the actual food would be a preferable source rather than synthetic vitamin A.

Tomatoes and Tomato Sauce:

Lycopene in tomatoes has proven to lead to longer survival for prostate cancer patients. Tomatoes also contain a whole series of anticancer nutrients whose combined action is more effective than lycopene on its own. If using canned tomato sauce, choose that in glass jars as plastic lined cans release BPA's. Of course sauce should not contain added sugar. We grow a lot of tomatoes every summer and the meaty ones can be halved and sprinkled with olive oil and a little sea salt or dried herbs and roasted at low temperature until most of the moisture has gone out of them and then put into freezer bags (place them in a single layer until frozen). They are delicious all winter in dishes that call for tomatoes. Cooked tomatoes are richer in lycopene and raw tomatoes are also rich in vitamin C. Tomatoes must be cooked to release lycopene and olive oil improves assimilation.

Soy:

Soy is a little bit controversial but Dr. Weil, Dr. Servan-Schreiber and others recommend it ORGANIC ONLY. Soy isoflavones include genistein, daidzein, and glycitein which block the stimulation of cancer cells by estrogens and testosterones. Note: Isoflavone pills have been shown to aggravate certain breast cancers but this is not so for soy taken as raw food. I have personally kept my soy intake minimal but do use soy "sour cream" and "cream cheese" sparingly.

Mushrooms:

Shitake, maitake, enokidake, cremini, portobello, oyster, and thistle oyster mushrooms all contain polysaccharides and lentinian, which stimulate the reproduction and activity of immune cells. Maitake probably has most pronounced effect on immune system. These are beginning to show up fresh and dried in supermarkets. I get them dried to use in soups, and sprinkle on salads.

Cilantro:
Chopped and sprinkled on salads and other dishes, this herb is very good for liver detoxification especially after exposure to radiation such as X-rays and scans. I try to put it in salads often. I've read in many different sources that it is also a chelate binding to aluminum, lead, mercury and such heavy metals we need to get out of our bodies. I also take a Red Desert Clay tablet (from www.Iamperfectlyhealthy.com) daily to clean up any toxic molecules the cilantro "drops".

Parsley and Celery:
Contain apigenin, an anti-inflammatory molecule that promotes apoptosis and blocks angiogenesis. Organic is really important in celery. It is usually the basis of my fresh vegetable juice. It juices well and counts as both nutraceutical and water.

Sea Vegetables (seaweed or algae):
Nori, Combu, Wakame, Arame, Dulse are commonly available dried sea vegetables carried by most supermarkets. Nori contains long chain omega-3 fatty acids– the most effective against inflammation. Kombu shortens cooking time for legumes and makes them more digestible. All these (algae) have plenty of nutraceutical chemicals and can be used in cooking. I prefer Dulse and keep it in a shaker on the table. These are bright colored vegetable flakes with phytochemicals in them.

Pomegranate Juice:
Some studies show that 8 ounces a day with breakfast has slowed the spread of an established prostate tumor by 67%. It's been used in Persian medicine for thousands of years and its anti-inflammatory and

antioxidant properties are confirmed. I eat pomegranates in season. There are good videos on YouTube demonstrating how to easily harvest the fruit inside them.

Plums, Peaches, Nectarines:
Recently, researchers discovered that these large stone fruit (especially plums) contain as many anti-cancer agents as berries and at far lower cost. A study at University of Texas showed plum extracts powerful against breast cancer.

Apples:
A good fruit (organic or peeled) that is a vitamin C source as well as a satisfying and cleansing snack, apples may well help "keep the doctor away" as Dr. Andrew Weil, M.D. has written in his eNewsletter (www.drweil.com) on several occasions.

Berries:
Strawberries, raspberries, blueberries, blackberries, and cranberries all contain elegiac acid and a large number of polyphenols. They stimulate the elimination of carcinogenic substances and inhibit angiogenesis. Anthocyanidins and proanthocyanidins in berries also promote apoptosis in cancer cells. Freezing does not damage the anticancer molecules in these berries so they can be used year round. They do not raise the blood levels of glucose, insulin and the (insulin growth factor) like most other fruits. They are great in a Budwig smoothie with yogurt, flax oil, and stevia. I eat a LOT of fresh and frozen berries - especially raspberries, blueberries, and strawberries (organic).

I also take Elderberry Extract capsules that have much the same nutrients as raspberries. I probably eat three cups of fresh or frozen berries a week and sometimes more.

To extend the refrigerator life of fresh strawberries, blueberries and raspberries, there are two products I use that seem to work in the refrigerator circulating ozone or oxygen which keeps down the organisms that "wilt" these fruits. One is called "Berry Breeze Activated Oxygen Fridge Freshener" and the other is called "03 Pure Fridge Deodorizer and Food Preserver". I have one of each and they both help keep produce fresher longer. They run on D or C batteries.

Appendix Three of this book provides a Food Nutraceutical Chart.

Herb and Spice Nutraceuticals:

A scientific overview of certain molecules in spices (and herbs) from Dr. Bharat B. Aggarwal, et al of the University of Texas M.D. Anderson Cancer Center, is available in a National Institute of Health manuscript entitled: "Molecular Targets of Nutraceuticals Derived from dietary Spices: Potential Role in suppression of Inflammation and Tumorigenesis (tumor growth)". Dr. Aggarwal is also the author of the book: *Healing Spices,* and he pioneered the work disclosing Turmeric/Curcumin as a powerful anti-cancer spice.

I quote from this report: "There is increasing evidence for the importance of plant-based foods in regular diet to lowering the risk of most chronic diseases, so spices are now emerging as more than just flavor aids, but as agents that can not only prevent but may even treat disease . . . Besides suppressing inflammatory pathways, spice-derived nutraceuticals can suppress survival, proliferation, invasion, and angiogenesis (blood vessel growth) of tumor cells."[24] Molecules in certain spices and herbs can also promote apoptosis or rogue cell suicide.

I believe the technicality of Aggarwal's manuscript illustrates the seriousness of the science, and the 223 research documents cited give it much credence. Even if you don't read the technical details, you can benefit from the useful graphs and charts. Several tables are included that identify the active molecules against specific cancer mechanisms starting with inflammation which we discussed at length earlier and expand in Appendix Five.

In Appendix Four of this book, I include a simplified summary compiled from this manuscript categorizing the information in the research tables to make a more useful quick reference.

Anti-oxidants:

Dark Chocolate:
Dark chocolate (more than 70% cocoa) contains a number of antioxidants, proanthocyanidins, and many polyphenols (a square of this chocolate contains twice as many of these anti-cancer molecules as a glass of red wine and almost as many as a cup of green tea steeped properly. WATCH FOR SUGAR CONTENT. Chocolate is unlikely to have the toxic additives required by law in red wine. Twenty grams of this chocolate a day is acceptable. Its glycemic index is markedly lower than white bread which I avoid. It can be melted over fruit. I use the 85% cocoa bars (organic) in moderation .

Selenium:
Selenium stimulates immune cells, especially NK (Natural Killer cells) by 80%, and boosts anti-oxidant mechanisms in the body.

Organic fruits and fish....especially wild caught salmon, tuna, sardines, trout etc.

Probiotics:
Organic yogurt or kefir (yogurt milk) from low temperature pasteurized milk is a good source. Commercial processed yogurt that has been high temperature pasteurized kills most of the probiotic organisms but still works in the Budwig smoothie.

The intestines ordinarily contain friendly bacteria, which helps digestion and facilitates regular bowel elimination. These bacteria also help stabilize the immune system. The most common are Lactobacillus acidophilus and Lactobacillus bifidus. It's been shown that these probiotics inhibit growth of cancer cells in the colon in more ways than just helping move matter out of the body regularly so that carcinogenic substances in food are not held for re-absorption. Studies show that probiotics improve the performance of immune system and increase the number of Natural

Killer Cells. On the advice of the naturopathic doctor I consulted, I take one tablet at bedtime of Dr. Ohhira's Probiotic.

Food Synergy - Combining Foods For Optimum Benefit

Online you can find helpful food combining charts at www.alderbrooke. com. The October 21, 2011 post on www.realhealthhope.com entitled "Food combinations - Working With Nature" shares directions I received from the naturopathic doctor I personally consulted.

Here I want to share from the book, *Foods to Fight Cancer,* regarding combining anticancer agents in food to increase their helpful activity. The authors, Beliveau and Gingras, say, "We have seen that the anticancer agents present in food are often capable of acting directly on a tumor and restricting its development by causing death of cancerous cells and by preventing the tumor from progressing to a more advanced stage . . . Researchers have found that combining foods with distinct anticancer compounds allows them to target different processes involved in tumor growth, as well as making their activity more effective." [25]

These researchers point out that curcumin combined with green tea is an example of "direct synergy" which enhances the anticancer impact on a cell beyond that of small amounts of either food eaten separately. Additionally, "indirect synergy" is also a positive factor in anticancer foods, and an example is adding piperine (present in black pepper) to curcumin that increases absorption by a factor of 1000. [26]

Many foods combined for flavor also have nutraceutical synergy like lemon and kale, tomatoes and avocados, blueberries and walnuts, etc. I want to make your aware of food synergy without listing stressful rules. It is critical that we enjoy what we eat. I think you will find great pleasure in knowing your eating is empowering your body to heal.

I've been compelled to use a few food extract supplements to assure consistency of synergistic nutraceutical intake.

Glyconutrients:

Glyconutrients are sugars. Yes, they are carbohydrates and we need carbohydrates in our diets. HOWEVER, sugar molecules differ in make up and function and some are essential and some can be lethal rather like the different fats.

Dr. Benjamin Carson, M.D. is a world-renowned surgeon and professor at Johns Hopkins University Medical School. Diagnosed with an aggressive prostate cancer in 2003, Dr. Carson shares his story openly regarding his use of glyconutrients.

As reported in an interview in "Dallas Weekly", February 2004, when making treatment decisions, Dr. Carson recalled a friend who had been given three months to live yet changed his diet and pursued proper nutrition. Carson says, "The friend was still around and doing well. As a result I started to look at nutritional supplements. Then the father of one of my patients told me about a ten year old company in Texas which had world-wide patent rights to a food supplement known as glyconutrients." Dr. Carson contacted the company and says he was surprised by the amount of science they provided saying, "I was impressed that they did not make any wild medical claims." He adds, "The science made sense to me. God gave us (in plants) what we need to remain healthy. In today's world our food chain is depleted of nutrients and our environment has helped destroy what God gave us."[27]

Dr. Carson supported his immune system with glyconutrients and shares that he almost immediately saw abatement in his condition. He is quoted as saying, "I began to think that I did not need to have surgery or any other type of treatment. I seriously considered not having any type of procedure. I thought I could beat the cancer by supporting my body through glyconutritional supplementation." Yet he eventually decided to have a medical procedure because of his concern for those who might emulate his decision even though they might not be as conscientious about taking the supplements as he was. He says, "Because of my experience with glyconutrients, I was able to return to work in three weeks." [28]

Dr. Carson does NOT claim that glyconutrients actually cured his cancer and their use was only part of his treatment protocol. He is interviewed on this subject on Youtube.[29]

❖ Glyconutrients are the 6 essential ones out of 200+ <u>mostly</u> plant based carbohydrates and they include:
❖ xylose– present in kelp, ground psyllium seeds
❖ fucose (not fructose)– present in human breast milk but also in certain seaweeds.
❖ galactose– present in the spice fenugreek and lots of other foods like apples and grapes as well as in Echinacea
❖ glucose– widely available in food
❖ mannose– present in aloe vera and fenugreek spice
❖ N-acetylglucosamine– present in human breast milk and shiitake mushrooms
❖ N-acetylgalactosamin– present in shiitake mushrooms
❖ N-acetylneuraminic acid– present in organic hens eggs and grass fed red meat

In the body they have anti-inflammatory and anti-allergic benefits. Some studies show they block liver lectins that mediate tumor metastasis and protect intestinal mucosa against disease and cancer promoting agents.

The molecular makeups of these essential sugars are important but beyond the scope of this book. Their function is to combine with other molecules like proteins to coat the surface of every cell in the human body and function in cell adhesion and communication.

They are not vitamins, minerals, or enzymes but exist and function uniquely. All the many trillions of cells in our bodies need them. Each enhances the function of all the others in proportions determined by our "design". Supplementing them is not "the silver bullet" but they are part of the nutrients our bodies require at the cellular level, which, of course, extends to the bodily level of health. Any supplementation should be a complex of them all because they work together.

These sugars guide the cellular communication that is essential for normal cell and tissue development and physiological function." [30]

Beta Glucan May be Nature's Secret Indeed

In contrast to the glyconutrients, I have been blogging about (and taking) Beta Glucan for years. You will find a label category on this subject on, www.realhealthhope.com. I am not an expert, but I've read much of the research done by Dr. Vaclav Vetvicka, PhD at the University of Louisville and summarized in his book, *Beta Glucan: Nature's Secret*.

Beta glucan is isolated from yeasts, mushrooms, algae, or cereal grains and binds to the surfaces of the immune system cells- specifically macrophages (that engulf invader cells) and Natural Killer Cells. Dr. Vetvicka writes in an article entitled "Fighting Cancer" on his website, www.glucan.us that "The result of this interaction is that the highly activated tumor killers circulate in our body and actively seek and destroy their preferred targets - cancer cells. Upon contact with these cancer cells, they kill them in a specific way, which means they destroy only the cancer cells and leave the surrounding tissues and organs remaining intact and unharmed." [31]

I continue quoting from Vetvicka's website regarding Beta Glucan's function; however, as always, I encourage you to consult with "the Great Physician" and your health care advisors in making your own treatment decisions. Dr. Vetvicka extends his earlier point: "However, the important effects of glucan do not end in activation of immunocytes (immune cells noted). Besides the ability to stimulate the cells of the immune system to perform optimally and maximally, beta glucan also "cares" about their numbers (immune system cells). It is well established that all cells involved in immune reactions originate from common precursors- stem cells originating in bone marrow, resulting in a more rapid flow of new immunocytes into the bloodstream and into the various lymphoid organs throughout the body. These effects are important not only under normal conditions, as the increased amount of immunocytes in circulation means increased surveillance against potential invaders, but particularly in case of extreme stress such as in cancer, where the limited influx is further reduced by exhaustion of the immune system and by treatments such as irradiation and chemotherapy."[32]

Dr. Vetvicka points out that the action described in the above paragraph "would be enough to consider beta glucan one of the most significant anti-cancerous immunostimulants we know, but it has another 'ace up its sleeve'." He describes Beta Glucan, once it enters the bloodstream, as activating cells to stimulate other defense systems "including tumor necrosis factor (TNF), interleukins 1 and 6, hydrogen peroxide, and gamma interferon "all of which are proven effective in our fight against cancers." He adds that the impact is systemic and fully arms the immune system. [33]

Dr. Vetvicka's research indicates dosage levels are important. I could find no indication that the research looking for toxicity in overdose disclosed any. There is indication that this glucan is beneficial against diseases other than cancer. For more information: www.transferpoint.com/research which is the manufacturer of the "brand" Cancer Crusader Bill Henderson recommends.[34]

Sprouted Seeds and Grains are Live Food

There are two blog posts on www.realhealthhope.com about sprouting seeds for food and using sprouted grains for baking. They are dated February 5, 2011 and February 12, 2013 respectively. [49]Sprouting makes it easy to grow considerable nutrition in one square foot of space year round. My favorite is broccoli sprouts, which are extremely easy to grow in a glass jar with a screen lid from organic sprouting seeds ordered online.

The process is simple. First cover jar bottom with a thin layer of broccoli sprouting seed and add two inches of filtered water. Soak the seeds overnight and rinse. I turn the jar almost upside down leaning on something and rinse them twice daily until they are about half an inch long. There are photos of my own sprouting efforts on the above cited blog posts. In about 3 days, there are enough sprouts to sprinkle over salads adding live electron rich nutrition. Sprouts are high in protein so I'm careful to pace intake. My grandchildren eat them like candy and I'm happy they are getting the anti-cancer molecule sulphoraphane. The sprouts contain 50 times more of this nutrient than mature broccoli.

Sprouted Grains in Cereal and Bread

I began eating Ezekiel 4:9 bread shortly after my "strike two surgery" and continue. I admit to occasionally eating a little whole wheat or rye bread, but for the first few years after surgery, I ate only sprouted organic bread. I use the "low glycemic index" type and keep a few loaves in the freezer. It thaws deliciously in a toaster and it's great for sandwiches or toast.

Ezekiel 4:9 brand is also available in sprouted grain pasta, tortillas and cereals sold frozen (except the cereal and pasta). I order sprouted grain and legume flours online from www.sproutedorganicflour.com.

Why sprouted? Again, I'm seeking the qualities of easily digestible "living food" with natural innate nutrients including enzymes. I don't want refined sugars, sodium chloride, lots of wheat gluten that converts immediately to sugar, and I don't want genetically modified food. Sprouting provides efficient protein including all 9 amino acids.

I've learned that good food may appear to cost more than "standard shelf fare" in a super market, but it provides considerably more "bang for the buck" because it is more satisfying, energizing, healing, and sustaining.

The enzymes in "living food" facilitate digesting them. We are born with a finite supply of enzymes and aren't really designed to use those for digesting foods in which enzymes are depleted by processing including high temperature cooking. Thus we have another rationale for including plenty of raw vegetables and some fruits in our diets. I also supplement with digestive enzyme - another important topic for prayer dialog.

Cooked Foods? It Sacrifices Enzymes

Throughout this book, I've stressed the importance of DAILY including a LOT of fresh vegetables (and some whole fruits) in our anticancer diet. For at least two years after my "strike two surgery", I kept my diet vegan (except Budwig Protocol) with at least 80% raw. I eat a few more cooked foods now, but I try to not cook the life out of vegetables and I eat no fried foods. I do some low temperature "stir frying" and "oven roasting". When I dry vegetables from the garden, I'm careful to keep the temperature below 115 degrees to protect enzymes.

Currently, I'm experimenting with vegan cooking using pure Indian spices because they are strongly anti-cancer and very tasty. Again, balance is key. Extremes, I believe, push us off the road of life into ditches that work against our wholeness.

Meat and Dairy? There are REAL Issues

After a couple of years eating a vegan diet (except Budwig Protocol), a source for locally and naturally grown grass fed meat, eggs, wild caught salmon and low temperature pasteurized dairy opened near my home. I worked a very small amount of these foods into my diet; however, I do NOT eat products from animals grown with added hormones and antibiotics including "farm raised" fish.

I recommend the books, *The China Study* and *Whole*, by Dr. T. Colin Campbell, PhD and *The Hallelujah Diet* by George Malkmus. Both make good cases for a plant-based diet. In particular, Campbell points out two things animal protein "throws a wrench into". One: "The blood levels of the hormone, 1,25D (vitamin D) are depressed both by consuming too much animal protein and too much calcium (as in dairy products). [35] Two: Increased intake of animal protein also enhances the production of insulin-like growth factor (IGF-1) and this enhances cancer cell growth." [36] These are merely two of many possible examples of animal protein's tendency to interfere with normal biochemistry.

Dr. Campbell also says, "The most impressive evidence favoring plant-based diets is the way that so many food factors and biological events are integrated to maximize health and minimize disease. Plant-based diets don't tinker with our biological intricacies unless we ingest tainted or poison plants."[37] Campbell's books are so comprehensively documented it compelled me to minimize my intake of animal protein. Only when I needed to regain significant muscle mass did I sense in my spirit the need for a very small amount of this protein in my diet.

I'm not writing this book to impose a diet upon you. I assure you, from experience, that your body will respond positively to what the Lord directs.

No Brainers We Cannot Ignore

Surely you know by now the obvious healthy choice on the following:

- ❖ alcoholic beverages
- ❖ soft drinks and sports drinks
- ❖ tobacco products
- ❖ caffeine ("Teechino" is an amazing replacement for coffee.)
- ❖ sugar and artificial sweeteners
- ❖ highly refined and processed foods
- ❖ white table salt (and any added salt in excess)
- ❖ bleached flour products
- ❖ illicit drugs and self medicating with prescription drugs
- ❖ synthetic vitamins
- ❖ mineral supplements taken arbitrarily
- ❖ dietary supplements containing sugar
- ❖ "energy booster" drinks– including "pink" ones
- ❖ pharmaceuticals not prescribed by your physician

I suggest that you ask your doctor and/or pharmacist to help you understand the goal of taking any pharmaceutical. Is it short term or long term? What will it do in your body? Is there a way to remedy the situation through lifestyle change rather than adding the chemical? Is it a cure or is it symptom management to merely change lab results? Ask "the Great Physician" if the pharmaceutical is His choice for your health.

Notes:

twelve

Slam the Door on Cancer? Really?

It is done! Everyday it is done! We know that healing is in the atoning work of Jesus. He said, "It is finished" from the cross. People say, however, "I don't see it 'finished'– I see cancer and other diseases increasing". We see statistical facts only when we aren't looking for THE TRUTH such as David's praise, which I have shared several times in this book:

> Bless the LORD, O my soul: and all that is within me, bless his holy name.
> Bless the LORD, O my soul, and forget not all his benefits: Who forgives all thy iniquities; who heals all thy diseases;
> Who redeems thy life from destruction; who crowns thee with loving kindness and tender mercies. (Psalms 103:1-4, NKJV)

Note the "present tense" herein and remember God is not bound by what we see or by time, but He bound Himself to His Word, as David again praises: *I will worship toward thy holy temple, and praise thy name for thy loving kindness and for thy truth:* ***for thou hast magnified thy word (some translations say "thy saying") above all thy name***. (Psalms 138:2, KJV)

God gave us laws (principles) and He promised to respect them, as we must in order to "be in health" . . . natural laws, scientific laws, and spiritual laws . . . and they are the SAME laws (principles) regardless of label. They are laws He spoke into Creation that is an ongoing process as quantum physics is disclosing in agreement with Scripture. He gave His Word and we can count on that. We must be able to count on the universe created by His "saying" or the universe would have no order.

All Healing is Miraculous!

From our umbilical cord dropping off shortly after birth to disappearance of a tumor, our body is designed to heal. Doctors may stabilize us physically or remove an obstacle to healing. Ministers may lead someone to deliverance or repentance facilitating physical healing. Neither profession actually "heals". A surgeon can cut and sew, but our innate design heals the wounds surgery necessitates.

Healing is a "built in mechanism". Health is in Christ's atonement and resurrection victory. He did it ALL. Yes, our bodies age in time, but leaving this world because of disease at any age is not God's intention or character as disclosed in His word. Healing and health is "natural" and intended; sickness and dis-ease is "un-natural" and intended only by the enemy of our souls. The mindset for healing to manifest is realizing, as Keith and Megan Provance write in the booklet, *Scriptural Confessions for Healing*, "I am not sick and trying to get healed. I am already healed, and sickness is trying to take hold in my body. But I won't let it. . . I am healed and made whole in the mighty name of Jesus." [1]

Within this book, I have sought to provide insightful glimpses into the mystery of "present tense" healing perpetually available within the design and laws (principles) God spoke into Creation. God's written Word and Rhema Word are alive and pertinent to every material and spiritual phenomenon. Healing occurs when we embrace His intention for us as He has spoken it.

We cannot know everything, but we can "have a heart for God" and match our intention to His which is to accept ALL that Christ Jesus secured. Believers becomes "powerful Believers" when their spirit, soul and body discern Christ's spirit, soul and body.

Whether you do or don't believe what I've shared in this book, please ask God what will enable you to "slam the door on cancer (indeed on disease) and lock it out of your life".

Please join in the continued discussion at www.slamthedooroncancer.com intended to sustain the encouragement. Our original blog: www.realhealthhope.com will also remain online. Please join me on these blogs, and please know that this book is "from my heart and may it go to your heart" (L. Beethoven).

May the Lord bless you and keep you,

May the Lord cause His face to shine upon you and give you PEACE!

Notes:

Endnotes

Introduction:
1 Ecclesia Bible Society, *The Voice Bible*, (TN: Thomas Nelson, 2012), 1436.

Chapter One:
1. Norman Cousins, *Anatomy of an Illness (as perceived by the Patient).* (New York: W.W. Norton & Co., 1979), 55.

2. Rev. Cheryl Schang, *Heal Them All.* (Florida: Xulon Press, 2005), 39.

3. Schang, *Heal Them All*, 102.

4. Gary Sinclair, *Your Empowering Spirit.* (Celebrate Life), 132.

5. Dr. Bruce Lipton, PhD, *The Biology of Belief,* (CA: Hay House, 2005), 37.

6. Lipton, *The Biology of Belief, xv.*

7. Lipton, *The Biology of Belief,* 37.

8. Lipton, *The Biology of Belief,* 42.

9. Cal Pierce, "Destroying Cancer", CD Teaching, www.healingrooms.com.

10. Henry W. Wright, *A More Excellent Way to Be in Health,* (PA: Whitaker House, 2009), 58.

11. Wright, *A More Excellent Way,* 16.

12. Wright, *A More Excellent Way,* 233.

Chapter Two

1. Schang, *Heal Them All*, 77.

2. Schang, *Heal Them All*, 78.

3. Ibid.

4. David Youngii Cho, *The Fourth Dimension, VOL I.* , (FL: Bridge-Logos, 1979), 1.

5. David Youngii Cho, *The Fourth Dimension*, 86.

6. David Youngii Cho, *The Fourth Dimension*, 87.

7. Ibid.

8. David Youngii Cho, *The Fourth Dimension*, 90.

9. Ibid.

10. David Youngii Cho, *The Fourth Dimension*, 87.

11. Patrick Kavanaugh, *Spiritual Lives of the Great Composers*, (MI: Zondervan, 1982), 27.

12. Dr. Bernie S. Siegel, M.D., *Love, Medicine, & Miracles.* (NY: Harper and Row, 1998), 50.

13. Bill Johnson, mentioned in many sermons available on www.ibetheltv.com and podcasts "Bethel Sermon of the Week".

Chapter Three

1. Henry Drummond, *Natural Law and The Spiritual World.* (The Gutenberg Project) http://www.gutenberg.org/files/23334/23334-h/23334-h.htm.

2. Jay W. Richards, *Money, Greed, and God.* (NY: HarperOne), 86.

3. Frank Viola, *From Eternity to Here Re-discovering the Ageless Purpose of God.* (CO: David C. Cook, 2009), Introduction.

4. Bono podcast interview with Frank Viola, 25 June, 2013, http://ptmin.pod-bean.com/feed/

5. Jill Jackson and Sy Miller, "Let There Be Peace On Earth", 1955.

6. Kris Vallotton, "Walking Out of Pain I and II", www.ibetheltv.com.

7. David Servan-Schreiber, M.D., PhD, *The Anti-Cancer: A New Way of Life* (NY: Viking, 2009),150-153.

8. Norman Cousins, *Anatomy of an Illness (as perceived by the Patient)*. (NY: W.W. Norton & Co., 1979), 55.

9. Brother Lawrence, *The Practice of the Presence of God,* The Gutenberg Project http://cgsorder.com/lawrencebretext04brola10.pdf.

10. Bill Johnson, Conference Presentation, FUSE Church, Knoxville, TN, 26 September 2013. (I was present for this teaching)

11. Dr. Bernie Siegel, *Love, Medicine, & Miracles*, x.

12. Dr. Bernie Siegel, *Love, Medicine, & Miracles*, xi.

13. Dr. Bruce Lipton, *Biology of Belief,* 106.

Chapter Four
1. Bill Johnson, "Compassion Leads to Miracles", podcast, July 14, 2013.

2. Bill Johnson, *Strengthen Yourself in the Lord,* (PA: Destiny Image Publishing, 2007), 45.

3. T. J. McCrossan, B.A. and B.D., *Healing and the Atonement,* ed. Dr. Roy Hicks and Dr. Kenneth E. Hagin (Tulsa: Faith Library Publications, 1982), 25.

4. Schang, *Heal Them All,* 61

5. T. J. McCrossan, B.A. and B.D., *Healing and the Atonement,* 63.

6. Schang, *Heal Them All,* 26.

7. Schang, *Heal Them All,* 26-27.

8. Ibid.

9. Joseph Prince, *Health and Wholeness Through Holy Communion,* (UK: Kingsway Communications, Ltd., 2000), 14.

10. Joseph Prince, *Health and Wholeness,* 13.

11. Dr. Bernie Siegel, *Love, Medicine, & Miracles,* 119.

12. Marilyn Hickey, "Eight Ways God Heals", CD teaching, www.marilynand-sarah.org.

13. Katie Souza, "Kingdom of the Son", www.expectedendministries.com.

14. Harold R. Eberle, *The Spiritual, Mystical, and Supernatural, 2nd Edition.* (WA: Worldcast Publishing, 2011), 310.

SECTION II

Chapter Five
1. Wright, *A More Excellent Way,* 308-312.

2. Dr. Johanna Budwig, *Cancer– The Problem and the Solution,* (Germany: Nexus GmbH, 2008), 22.

3. Dr. Johanna Budwig, *Cancer,* 28.

4. Dr. Candace Pert, PhD, *Molecules of Emotion (Why You Feel the Way You Feel),* (NY: Scribner, 1997), 21.

5. Dr. Candace Pert, *Molecules of Emotion,* 242.

6. Dr. Candace Pert, *Molecules of Emotion,* 323.

7. Dr. Candace Pert, *Molecules of Emotion,* 25.

8. David Servan-Schreiber, M.D., PhD, *The Anti-Cancer Lifestyle,* 42.

9. Dr. Candace, Pert, PhD with Nancy Marriott. *Everything You Need to Know to Feel Go(od.* (CA: Hay House, Inc, 2006), 48.

Chapter Six
1. Masuru Emoto, *The Hidden Messages in Water,* trans. David A Thayne (NY: Atria Books/Beyond Words Publishing, Inc. 2001), 143.

2. Lipton, *The Biology of Belief*, 115.

3. Lipton, *The Biology of Belief*, 117.

4. David Van Koevering, *Your Keys to Taking Your Quantum Leap*, (TN: Elsewhen Research, 2007), 12.

5. David Van Koevering, *Your Keys*, 13.

6. Annette Capps, *Quantum Faith*, (England: Capps Publishing Co., 2003), 16.

7. Cal Pierce, "Healing, The Process to Establish Divine Health". Message given at Bethel Church, Redding, CA 22 June 2003.

8. David Van Koevering, *Your Keys*, 5.

9. Gary Sinclair, *Your Empowering Spirit*, 35.

10. Gary Sinclair, *Your Empowering Spirit*, 35

11. Gary Sinclair, *Your Empowering Spirit*, 37.

Chapter Seven

1. Masuru Emoto, *The Hidden Messages*, 5 &13.

2. Henry W. Wright, "Healing Theology", CD Teaching, www.beinhealth.com.

3. Gary Sinclair, *Your Empowering Spirit*, 58.

4. David Youngii Cho, *The Fourth Dimension*, 51.

5. Ibid.

6. Charles Capps, *God's Creative Power*, (England: Capps Publishing Co., 2003), 17.

7. Ibid.

8. Bill Johnson,. "Making Demons Homeless", Bethel Church Sermon of the Week Podcast 8 September 2013. www.ibeheltv.com.

9. Charles Capps, *God's Creative Power*, 19.

10. Charles Capps, *God's Creative Power,* 92-93.

11. Charles Capps, *God's Creative Power,* 95.

12. Anita Siddiki, "Obtaining Your Healing", CD Series, www.wisdomministries.org.

13. Dodie Osteen, *Healed of Cancer.* (TX: Lakewood Church, 2003), 7.

14. Dodie Osteen, *Healed of Cancer,* 26-27.

15. Dr. Caroline Leaf, PhD, *Who Switched Off My Brain?, Revised* (Southlake, Texas: IMPROV Ltd., 2009) www.drleaf.com, 39.

16. Ibid.

17. Ibid.

18. Ibid.

19. Dr. Caroline Leaf, PhD, *Who Switched Off,* 40-43.

20. Henry Drummond, *Natural Law in the Spiritual World,* (Gutenberg Project), http://www.gutenberg.org/files/23334/23334-h/23334-h.htm, preface.

21. David Van Koevering, *Your Keys,* 3.

22. Dr. Caroline Leaf, PhD, *Who Switched Off,* 54.

23. Dr. Caroline Leaf, PhD, *Who Switched Off,* 53.

24. Ibid.

25. Dr. Caroline Leaf, PhD, *Who Switched Off,* 21.

26. Harold R. Eberle, *The Spiritual, Mystical, and Supernatural, 2nd Edition.* (WA: Worldcast Publishing, 2011), 138-139.

SECTION III

Chapter Eight

1. Anita Siddiki, "Obtaining Your Healing".

2. Bill Johnson, "God's Sovereignty and Our Responsibility", Bethel Church Sermon of the Week, 11August, 2013.

3. Norman Cousins, *Anatomy of an Illness,* 163.

4. Henry W. Wright, *A More Excellent Way,* 73.

5. Henry W. Wright, *A More Excellent Way,* 74.

6. Lipton, *The Biology of Belief,* 71.

7. Stephanie Mills and Nicolas Ashford, "Reach Out and Touch Somebody's Hand", (London: EMI Publisher, 1970).

8. Dr. Caroline Leaf, PhD, *Who Switched Off,* 147.

9. Ruth Sackman, *Re-thinking Cancer,* (NY: Square One Publishers, 2003), *66.*

10. Shane Ellison, "NEW! This Sleep Pill Stops Cancer?", *The People's Chemist* eNewsletter, 8 March 2013.

11. Dr. David Speigel, PhD, "How Sleep Fights Cancer", *The Daily Mail, www. dailymail.co.uk/health/article-198096/How-**sleep**-fight-**cancer**.html*

12. Dr. William Dement, M.D., PhD and Christopher Vaughan, *The Promise of Sleep.* (NY: Dell, 1999), 268-269.

13. Dr. William Dement, M.D., PhD and Christopher Vaughan, *The Promise of Sleep,* 269.

14. Heather L. Papinchak, et al., "Effectiveness of Houseplants in Reducing the Indoor Air Pollutant Ozone," *Hort Technology,* April-June 2009, 19(2): 286-290, http://horttech.ashspublications.org/content/19/2/286.full.pdf. Re-posted on www.renegadehealth.com March 25, 2013.

Chapter Nine
1. Lipton, *The Biology of Belief,* 51-53.

2. Lipton, *The Biology of Belief,* 60.

3. Dr. Johanna Budwig, *Flax Oil as True Aid,* (Vancouver: Apple Publishing, 1992), *6.*

4. Gary Gordon, M.D., D.O. with Herb Joiner-Bey, N.D., *The Omega-3 Miracle.* (CA: Freedom Press, 2004), 18&19.

5. Gary Gordon, M.D., D.O. with Herb Joiner-Bey, N.D., *The Omega-3 Miracle,* 21.

6. Warburg Biography by Richard A. Brand, M.D. at http://www.ncbi.nlm.nih.gov/pmc/articles/PMC2947689/

7. Dr. Johanna Budwig, *Cancer, the Problem and Solution,* (Germany: Nexus GmbH), 41.

8. Dr. Johanna Budwig, *Flax Oil as True Aid,* 54.

9. Dr. Johanna Budwig, *Flax Oil as True Aid,* 55

10. Dr. Richard N. Firshein, D.O., *The Nutraceutical Revolution.* (NY: Riverhead Books, 1998), 37.

11. Dr. Richard N. Firshein, D.O., *The Nutraceutical Revolution* , 40.

12. Bill Henderson, *Cancer-Free– Your Guide to Gentle, Non-toxic Healing, 2nd edition.* (Bradenton, FL: Booklocker.com, Inc., 2007), 99.

13. Dr. Steve Blake, *Vitamins & Minerals Demystified: A Self Teaching Guide.* (NY: McGraw-Hill, Inc., 2008), 99.

14. Dr. Steve Blake, *Vitamins & Minerals,* 101-102.

15. Dr. Johanna Budwig, *Flax Oil as True Aid,* 53.

16. Dr. Johanna Budwig, *Flax Oil as True Aid,* 54.

17. Shane Ellison, www.thepeopleschemist.com.

18. Shane Ellison, *Over-The-Counter Natural Cures,* (Naperville, IL: Sourcebooks, Inc, 2009), 5.

19. Ibid.

20. Shane Ellison, *Over-The-Counter,* 159.

21. Ibid.

22. Dr. Johanna Budwig, *Flax Oil as True Aid, 53.*

23. Henry W. Wright, *A More Excellent Way, 233.*

24. Shane Ellison, *Over-The-Counter,* 31.

25. Bill Henderson, Beating Cancer Gently eNewsletter, 30 November 2011, http://www.beating-cancer-gently.com/184nl.html

26. Dr. Andrew Weil, M.D., eNewsletter, 20 July 2009, www.drweil.com

27. Norman Cousins, *Anatomy of an Illness,* 88.

Chapter Ten

1. Fereydoon Batmanghelidj, M.D., *Water: For Health, for Healing, for Life,* (NY: Warner Books, 2003), 2.

2. Fereydoon Batmanghelidj, M.D., *Water: For Health,* 5.

3. Fereydoon Batmanghelidj, M.D., *Water: For Health,* 3.

4. Fereydoon Batmanghelidj, M.D., *Water: For Health,* 17.

5. Ibid.

6. Dr. Arthur C. Guyton, M.D. and Dr. John E. Hall, PhD, *The Textbook of Medical Physiology, eleventh edition,* (PA: Elsevier Saunders, 2006), 362.

7. Fereydoon Batmanghelidj, M.D., *Water: For Health,* 37.

8. Fereydoon Batmanghelidj, M.D., *Water: For Health,* 61.

9. Fereydoon Batmanghelidj, M.D., *Water: For Health,* 61-69.

10. Fereydoon Batmanghelidj, M.D., *Water: For Health,* 72.

11. Dr. Andrew Weil, M.D., "Best Bottled Water?", *Bulletin* 3 March 2010. www.drweil.com.

Chapter Eleven

1. Marilyn Hickey, *Be Healed,* (Englewood, CO: Marilyn Hickey Ministries, 2008), 41.

2. Blake, Dr. Steve, *Vitamins & Minerals Demystified: A Self Teaching Guide.* (NY: McGraw-Hill, 2008), 58-62.

3. Dr. Johanna Budwig, *Cancer: The Problem and the Solution.*, 34.

4. Dr. Candace Pert, *Everything You Need,* 71-75 .

5. Dr. Candace Pert, *Everything You Need,* 72.

6. Ibid.

7. Dr. Candace Pert, *Everything You Need,* 74.

8. Dr. Candace Pert, *Everything You Need,* 75.

9. Ibid.

10. Shane Ellison, http://thepeopleschemist.com/splenda-the-artificial-sweetener-that-explodes-internally/

11. Ibid.

12. Ibid.

13. Dr. Patrick Quillin, PhD, R.D., C.N.S, with Noreen Quillin, *Beating Cancer With Nutrition,* (CA: Nutrition Times Press, Inc., 1998), 139.

14. Dr. Andrew Weil, M.D., *Natural Health, Natural Medicine, Revised Edition,* (NY: Houghton Mifflin Co, 2004), 15.

15. Dr. David Servan-Schreiber, M.D., PhD., *Anticancer: A New Way of Life,* 65.

16. Dr. David Servan-Schreiber, M.D., PhD., *Anticancer,* 66.

17. Dr. David Servan-Schreiber, M.D., PhD., *Anticancer,* 68.

18. Dr. Andrew Weil, M.D. http://www.drweil.com/drw/u/QAA400590/Is-Honey-Healthy.html.

19. Colleen Story, "How Cinnamon could Help Treat and Prevent Type II Diabetes– Real Evidence. 27 September 2013, http://renegadehealth.com/blog/2013/09/27/how-cinnamon-could-help-treat-and-prevent-type-ii-diabetes-real-evidence.

20. Dr. Richard Beliveau, PhD and Dr. Denis Gingras, PhD, *Foods to Fight Cancer,* (NY: DK Publishing, 2007), 48-54.

21. Dr. David Servan-Schreiber, M.D., PhD., *Anticancer,* 105-108, and "Anticancer Action" Insert, 3-16.

22. Dr. Michail J. Wargovich, M.D., "The Cancer Bulletin", 376:1 (1985): 3-4.

23. Neev M. Arnell, "The Health Benefits of Phytochemicals", http://www.naturalnews.com/032463_phytochemicals_health_benefits.html .

24. Dr. Bharat B. Aggarwal, PhD, et al. "Molecular Targets of Nutraceuticals Derived from Dietary Spices: Potential Role in Suppression of Inflammation and Tumorigenesis", http://www.ncbi.nlm.nih.gov/pmc/articles/PMC3141288/pdf/nihms307487.pdf, abstract of Manuscript, 1.

25. Dr. Richard Beliveau, PhD and Dr. Denis Gingras, PhD, *Foods to Fight Cancer,* (NY: DK Publishing, 2007), 176

26. Dr. Richard Beliveau, PhD and Dr. Denis Gingras, PhD, *Foods,* 178.

27. Dr. Benjamin Carson, M.D., quoted in Dallas Weekly Magazine, February 2004, http://www.cell-to-cell-health.com/support-files/drbscarson.pdf.

28. Ibid.

29. Dr. Benjamin Carson, M.D., "Integrative Medicine" interview, http://youtu.be/o0goWh9aosY

30. Ram Sasisekharan, PhD and James R. Myette (MIT), "The Sweet Science of Glycobiology: Complex carbohydrates, molecules that are particularly important for communication among cells, are coming under systematic study". *American Scientist, Vol 91,* (2003), www.americanscientist.org

31. Dr. Vaclav Vetvicka, PhD. "Fighting Cancer", www.glucan.us.

32. Ibid.

33. Ibid.

34. Bill Henderson, *Cancer-Free– Your Guide to Gentle, Non-toxic Healing, 2nd ed.*, 89.

35. Dr. T. Colin Campbell, PhD and Thomas M. Campbell. *The China Study.* (TX: Benbella Books, 2006), 364.

36. Dr. T. Colin Campbell, PhD and Thomas M. Campbell. *The China Study*, 365.

37. Dr. T. Colin Campbell, PhD and Thomas M. Campbell. *The China Study*, 361.

Chapter Twelve
1. Keith and Megan Provance, *Scriptural Confessions for Healing Gift Collection.* (Tulsa, OK: Harrison House, 2007), 12.

Appendix One

Healing Word of God

Exodus 15:26 (NKJV) *If you diligently heed the voice of the LORD your God and do what is right in His sight, give ear to His commandments and keep all His statutes, I will permit none of the diseases on you which I have brought on the Egyptians. For I am the LORD who heals you.*

Exodus 23:25 (NKJV) *You shall serve the LORD your God, and He will bless your bread and your water. And He will take sickness away from the midst of you.*

Deuteronomy 7:15 (NKJV) *The LORD will take away from you all sickness, and will afflict you with none of the terrible diseases of Egypt which you have known, but will lay them on all those who hate you.*

Deuteronomy 30:19 (NKJV) *I call heaven and earth as witnesses today against you, that I have set before you life and death, blessing and cursing; therefore choose life, that both you and your descendants may live.*

Joshua 21:45 (NKJV) *Not a word failed of any good thing, which the LORD had spoken to the house of Israel. All came to pass.*

Psalms 30:2 (KJV) *O Lord my God, I cried unto thee, and thou hast healed me. Even to the dividing asunder of soul and spirit.*

Psalms 42:11 (KJV) *Why art thou cast down, O my soul? And why art thou disquieted within me? Hope thou in God: for I shall yet praise him, who is the health of my countenance, and my God.*

Psalms 91:10-11 (ASV) *There shall no evil befall thee, Neither shall any plague come nigh thy tent. For He will give his angels charge over thee, to keep thee in all thy ways.*

Psalms 91:16 (NKJV) *With long life I will satisfy him, and show him My salvation.*

Psalms 103:1-5 (NKJV) *Bless the LORD, O my soul; And all that is within me, bless His holy name. Bless the LORD, O my soul, And forget not all His benefits: Who forgives all your iniquities, Who heals all your diseases, Who redeems your life from destruction, Who crowns you with loving kindness and tender mercies, Who satisfies your mouth with good things, So that your youth is renewed like the eagle's.*

Psalms 107:20 (KJV) ***He*** *sent His word and healed them, And delivered them from their destructions.*

Psalms 118:17 (NKJV) *I shall not die, but live, And declare the works of the LORD.*

Proverbs 4:20-22 (NKJV) *My son, give attention to my words; Incline your ear to my sayings. Do not let them depart from your eyes; Keep them in the midst of your heart. For they are life to those who find them, and health to all their flesh.*

Proverbs 4:22 (KJV) *For they (His Words) are life unto those that find them, and health to all their flesh.*

Proverbs 12:18 (ASV) *There is that speaks rashly like the piercings of a sword; But the tongue of the wise is health.*

Isaiah 43:25-26 (NKJV) *I am He who blots out your transgressions for My own sake; And I will not remember your sins. Put Me in remembrance; Let us contend together;* ***State your case****, that you may be acquitted.*

Isaiah 53:5 (NKJV) *He was wounded for our transgressions, He was bruised for our iniquities; The chastisement for our peace was upon Him, And by His stripes we* are *healed.*

Isaiah 55:11 *The Word of God will accomplish what it was sent out to do.*

Jeremiah 30:17 (NKJV) *I will restore health to you And heal you of your wounds, says the LORD, 'Because they called you an outcast saying: "This is Zion; No one seeks her."*

Joel 3:10 (NKJV) *Let the weak say, 'I am strong'.*

Nahum 1:7 (KJV) *The LORD is good, a strong hold in the day of trouble; and he knows them that trust in Him.*

Nahum 1:9 (NKJV) *Your sickness will leave and not come back again. What do you conspire against the LORD? He will make an utter end of it. Affliction will not rise up a second time.*

Malachi 3:10 (NKJV) *Bring all the tithes into the storehouse, That there may be food in My house, And try Me now in this, Says the LORD of hosts, If I will not open for you the windows of heaven And pour out for you such blessing That there will not be room enough to receive it.*

Malachi 4:2 (KJV) *But unto you that fear my name shall the Sun of righteousness arise with healing in his wings; and ye shall go forth, and grow up as calves of the stall.*

Matthew 8:2-3 (NKJV) *Behold, a leper came and worshipped Him, saying, "Lord, if You are willing, You can make me clean. Then Jesus put out His hand and touched him, saying, "I am willing; be cleansed." Immediately his leprosy was cleansed.*

Matthew 8:17 (KJV) *When the even was come, they brought unto him many that were possessed with devils: and he cast out the spirits with his word, and healed all that were sick: that it might be fulfilled which was spoken by Esaias (Isaiah) the prophet, saying, Himself took our infirmities, and bare our sicknesses.*

Matthew 18:18 (NKJV) *I say to you, whatever you bind on earth will be bound in heaven, and whatever you loose on earth will be loosed in heaven.*

Matthew 18:19 (NKJV) *I say to you that if two of you agree on earth concerning anything that they ask, it will be done for them by My Father in heaven.*

Mark 11:22-23 (NKJV) *So Jesus answered and said to them, "Have faith in God. "For assuredly, I say to you, whoever **says** to this mountain, 'Be removed and be cast into the sea,' and does not doubt in his heart, but believes that those things he **says** will be done, he will have whatever he **says**."*

Mark 11:24 (NKJV) *I say to you, whatever things you ask when you pray, believe that you receive them, and you will have them*

Mark 16:17 (ASV) *And these signs shall accompany them that believe: in my name shall they cast out demons; they shall speak with new tongues;*

Luke 13:11-13, 16 (KJV) *And, behold, there was a woman which had a spirit of infirmity eighteen years, and was bowed together, and could in no wise lift up herself. And when Jesus saw her, he called her to him, and said unto her, Woman, thou art loosed from thine infirmity. And he laid his hands on her: and immediately she was made straight, and glorified God.* **(16)** *And ought not this woman, being a daughter of Abraham, whom Satan hath bound, lo, these eighteen years, be loosed from this bond on the sabbath day?*

John 9:31 (NKJV) *We know that God does not hear sinners; but if anyone is a worshiper of God and does His will, He hears him.*

John 10:10 (NKJV) *The thief does not come except to steal, and to kill, and to destroy. I have come that they may have life, and that they may have it more abundantly.*

John 14:12-14 (KJV) *Verily, verily, I say unto you, He that believes on me, the works that I do shall he do also; and greater works than these shall he do; because I go unto my Father. And whatsoever ye shall ask in my name, that will I do, that the Father may be glorified in the Son. If ye shall ask any thing in my name, I will do it.*

Acts 10:38 (KJV) *How God anointed Jesus of Nazareth with the Holy Ghost and with power: who went about doing good, and healing all that were oppressed of the devil; for God was with him.*

Romans 8:2 *For the law of the Spirit of life in Christ Jesus hath made me free from the law of sin and death.*

Romans 8:11 (NKJV) *But if the Spirit of Him who raised Jesus from the dead dwells in you, He who raised Christ from the dead will also give life to your mortal bodies through His Spirit who dwells in you.*

1 Corinthians 6:19-20 (ASV) *Or know ye not that your body is a temple of the Holy Spirit which is in you, which ye have from God? And ye are not your own; for ye were bought with a price: glorify God therefore in your body.*

2 Corinthians 1:20 (NKJV) *All the promises of God in Him are Yes, and in Him Amen, to the glory of God through us.*

2 Corinthians 5:21 (AMP) *For our sake He made Christ [virtually] to be sin Who knew no sin, so that in and through Him we might become [endued with,* *viewed as being in, and examples of] the righteousness of God [what we ought to be, approved and acceptable and in right relationship with Him, by His goodness].*

2 Corinthians 10:4-5 (NKJV) *Cast down those thoughts and imaginations that don't line up with the Word of God. For the weapons of our warfare are not carnal but mighty in God for pulling down strongholds, casting down arguments and every high thing that exalts itself against the knowledge of God, bringing every thought into captivity to the obedience of Christ,*

Galatians 2:20 (KJV) *I am crucified with Christ: nevertheless I live; yet not I, but Christ lives in me: and the life which I now live in the flesh I live by the faith of the Son of God, who loved me, and gave himself for me.*

Galatians 3:13-14 (NKJV) *Christ has redeemed us from the curse of the law, having become a curse for us (for it is written, "Cursed is everyone who hangs on a tree"), that the blessing of Abraham might come upon the Gentiles in Christ Jesus, that we might receive the promise of the Spirit through faith.*

Ephesians 6:10-17(NKJV) *be strong in the Lord's power. Put on His armor to fight for healing. Finally, my brethren, be strong in the Lord and in the power of His might. Put on the whole armor of God, that you may be able to stand against the wiles of the devil. For we do not wrestle against flesh and blood, but against principalities, against powers, against the rulers of the darkness of this age, against spiritual hosts of wickedness in the heavenly places. Therefore take up the whole armor of God, that you may be able to withstand in the evil day, and having done all, to stand. Stand therefore, having girded your waist with truth, having put on the breastplate of righteousness, and having shod your feet with the preparation of the gospel of peace; above all, taking the shield of faith with which you will be able to quench all the fiery darts of the wicked one. And take the helmet of salvation, and the sword of the Spirit, which is the word of God.*

Philippians 2:13 (KJV) *For it is God which works in you both to will and to do of his good pleasure.*

Colossians 1:12 (AMP) *Giving thanks to the Father, Who has qualified and made us fit to share the portion, which is the inheritance of the saints (God's holy people) in the Light.*

2 Timothy 1:7 (NKJV) *Fear is not of God. Rebuke it! For God has not given us a spirit of fear, but of power and of love and of a sound mind.*

Hebrews 4:12 *For the word of God is quick and powerful, and sharper than any two-edged sword.*

Hebrews 10:23 (NKJV) *You will not waiver in your faith. Let us hold fast the confession of our hope without wavering, for He who promised is faithful.*

Hebrews 10:35 (NKJV) *Therefore do not cast away your confidence, which has great reward.*

Hebrews 13:8 (NKJV) *Jesus Christ is the same yesterday, today, and forever.*

James 1:21 (ASV) *Wherefore putting away all filthiness and overflowing of wickedness, receive with meekness the implanted word, which is able to save your souls."*

James 5:14-15 (NKJV) *Is anyone among you sick? Let him call for the elders of the church, and let them pray over him, anointing him with oil in the name of the Lord. And the prayer of faith will save the sick, and the Lord will raise him up. And if he has committed sins, he will be forgiven."*

1 Peter 2:24 (NKJV) *He Himself bore our sins in His own body on the tree, that we, having died to sins, might live for righteousness; by whose stripes you were healed.*

1 Peter 5:8-9 (KJV) *Be sober, be vigilant; because your adversary the devil, as a roaring lion, walks about, seeking whom he may devour: Whom resist steadfast in the faith, knowing that the same afflictions are accomplished in your brethren that are in the world.*

1 John 3:21-22 (NKJV) *If our heart does not condemn us, we have confidence toward God. And whatever we ask we receive from Him, because we keep His commandments and do those things that are pleasing in His sight.*

1 John 4:4 (ASV) *Ye are of God, my little children, and have overcome them: because greater is he that is in you than he that is in the world.*

1 John 5:14-15 (NKJV) *Now this is the confidence that we have in Him, that if we ask anything according to His will, He hears us. And if we know that He hears us, whatever we ask, we know that we have the petitions that we have asked of Him.*

3 John 1:2 (KJV) *Beloved, I wish above all things that thou may prosper and be in health, even as thy soul prospers.*

Revelation 12:11 NKJV *And they overcame him by the blood of the Lamb and by the word of their testimony, and they did not love their lives to the death.*

Sources and References

Scripture and Faith Building Books:
I have put these in an order of emphasis not because any on the list are not helpful but because I know that time may be of the essence to my readers:

*****The Holy Bible*
I recommend you invest in a good Word Study Concordance and/or a Young's Literal Translation and/or a Greek Interlinear New Testament and/or use good Bible software like www.bluewordbible.com or www.biblegateway.com (these are free) or the one I use (not free), WordSearch. [Note: Of course there is Biblical narrative (such as in the book of Job) in the Bible that, while true, are not "truth" or the basis for doctrine and context is important for realizing the layers of truth in God's Word. I urge you to pray for insight and discernment of the Word as you read.]

****Heal Them All* by Rev. Cheryl Schang
Easy to read, theologically sound, totally encouraging. I wish I had found it sooner. This book will help you understand Scripture regarding healing.

****God's Creative Power for Healing* by Charles Capps
This comes in pamphlet/booklet or a nice bonded leather "pocket book". I have used this book to turn back relapse "attacks". ESSENTIAL! Read it like taking medicine.

***Health and Wholeness Through The Holy Communion* and *Right Believing* by Joseph Prince. These two books offer VERY Important insights. Life saving discernment!

***Healing Bible Study* by Kenneth E Hagin

This book, with the Bible, saved my life. Don't be afraid of this book even if your "church denomination" doesn't study Hagin. His own testimony is woven throughout this book and it is a faith-building dynamo. Remember, "We overcome by the blood of the lamb and the word of our testimony." (Rev. 12:11)

***Release the Power of Jesus and Strengthen Yourself in the Lord* (2 books) by Bill Johnson
Any of Johnson's books are beyond description for building Biblical faith. Every sentence is rich and anointed. His teaching is so sensitive to Holy Spirit and so practical for life that I really cannot describe the impact. Bill Johnson is lead pastor at Bethel Church, Redding, CA.

***The Hidden Messages in Water* by Masuru Emoto
Great insights that do not conflict with Scripture or Science. Includes amazing photographs. This book has meant a great deal to me.

***The Essential Guide to Healing* by Randy Clark and Bill Johnson
The title says it all. These pastors have powerful healing ministries all over the world. I believe you will find this book helpful for yourself and for ministering to others after you have returned to health.

**Bodily Healing and The Atonement* by T.J. McCrossan (reprint edited by K. Hagin and R. Hicks). It is absolutely true to the original book (which I have) of this renowned Greek scholar and minister, TJ McCrossan.

**Christ the Healer* by F.F. Bosworth. Classic and profound series of messages.

**Jesus Manifesto* by Leonard Sweet and Frank Viola.
An insightful disclosure of Jesus Christ. A "must read" because seeking the Healer is to seek health.

**Healed of Cancer* by Dodie Osteen.
Healing Scriptures and an amazing testimony.

**Be Healed* by Marilyn Hickey
This book served me well early in my search.

**Healing Scriptures* by Kenneth E. Hagin
I am not sure where I would be without this man's faith building and soundly Scriptural teaching to say nothing of his own testimony.

**Be Healed in Jesus' Name* by Joyce Meyer
A book of healing Scriptures with notes.

**Quantum Faith* by Annette Capps
A simple but sound explanation of quantum physics and its impact on faith that is very sound Scripturally.

**Keys to Taking Your Quantum Leap* by David Van Koevering
This book has a good bibliography but Dr. Van Koevering is a Christian physicist with a powerful personal healing testimony. He brings the physical and spiritual together in a way, I believe, anyone can understand it. He applies it to healing with great insight.

**Quantum Healing* and *Quantum Prayer* by Becky and David Van Koevering

**The Fourth Dimension* by David (Paul) Youngii Cho
Good book on praying effectively and faith building. I share his prayer teaching in the book.

**The Meal that Heals* by Perry Stone
Important teaching about Holy Communion!

Your Empowering Spirit by Gary Sinclair
This can be downloaded free online. Sinclair is a Christian who teaches soul awareness for healing. He has a strong personal testimony of healing from severe MS and congenital lung malformation.

Real Faith for Healing by Charles S. Price
A life changing book by one of "God's Generals". Classically written.

Insights into Cancer by Henry W. Wright
(He is also author of long time best seller *A More Excellent Way to Be in Health*, a compilation of lectures). www.beinhealth.com Wright deals with Spiritual and science.

Prison to Praise and *From Fear to Faith* (two books) by Merlin Coruthers
Life changing content. Coruthers was a WWII Paratrooper, aide to Eisenhower, and Army Chaplain

The Extraordinary Healing Power of Ordinary Things by Larry Dossey, M.D.
An encouraging book in a conversational way.

These and more resources are listed on my blogs:
www.slamthedooroncancer.com and www.realhealthhope.com.

Other Faith Building Resources:
"Healing School" by Katie Souza of www.expectedendministries.com. Katie offers some of her teachings "free" on the website link cited here. She also has an extraordinary testimony. I highly recommend her teaching, "How to Stay Un-Offendable" and "Pick Up Your Mat" but all of her teaching is foundational for lasting health.

"Obtaining Your Healing" (recorded teaching) by Dr. Nasir Siddicki and Anita Siddicki who both have extraordinary personal healing testimonies. www.widsomministries.org .

"Eight Ways God Heals", a CD teaching by Marilyn Hickey www.marilynandsarah.com.

Many resources at www.ibetheltv.com. Regardless of your "church home", I highly recommend you subscribe to the free podcasts of the weekly sermons from Bethel Church, Redding, CA. The live streams of their services are also amazing and the worship is highly anointed. You WILL be equipped and empowered.

Books with Scientific Information and Focus:
These are not necessarily in an order of significance but I have starred a few that have been particularly helpful to me.

Questioning Chemotherapy by Ralph W. Moss PhD. Note: I'm amazed that people rush into this option while still "in shock" and often while recovering from major surgery and without a second opinion or any reasonable idea what chemotherapy actually is, does, and does NOT do. It's the same with radiation. There are questions patients should ask.

Cancer Therapy: The Independent Consumer's Guide to Non-Toxic Treatment and Prevention by Ralph W. Moss PhD. Moss began his career as a medical reporter and continues it as an independent investigative reporter focusing on cancer.

Cancer-Gate by Samuel S. Epstein, M.D. This doctor explains what the cancer industry doesn't want the public to know about the success rates and long-term effects of treatment.

Death by Medicine by Dr. Gary Null, PhD with Dr. Martin Feldman, M.D., Dr. Debora Rasio, M.D. and Dr. Carolyn Dean, M.D., N.D. Information we should know for making treatment and health care choices– not a bashing of medical science but an objective view.

**Doctors Are More Harmful Than Germs* by Dr. Harvey Bigelsen, M.D. I thought the title "unfortunate" because it will probably keep many doctors from reading the book; however, Bigelsen, a surgeon, writes sensitively and candidly and explains a great deal about why no surgery is minor or routine. His insights into inflammation, I thought, provided critical information not found elsewhere. I wish I had this information 50 years ago. This is not a caustic or bitter book but one of compassion.

***Cure or Cover Up?* by Henry W. Wright offers important insights into pharmaceuticals.

Malignant Medical Myths by Joel M. Kaufman, Ph.D. Helpful in understanding how the cancer industry uses statistics. I didn't agree with a few of his personal opinions, but his factual reviews are sound and difficult to find in print.

***Flax Oil as a True Aid Against Arthritis, Heart Infarction, Cancer and other Diseases* by Dr. Johanna Budwig. Don't let the funky title fool you. You may find this book online free in pdf. VERY important information but harder to read than Dr. Budwig's other book (below).

****Cancer: The Problem and the Solution* by Dr. Johanna Budwig. This book, using the previously "missing link" of quantum physics regarding solar photons, explains Budwig's extension of Dr. Otto Warburg's Nobel Prize winning work regarding cellular level energy generation and how the flax oil/protein diet delivers the necessary electrons. VERY IMPORTANT!

***The China Study* and *Whole* (2 books) by T. Colin Campbell, PhD. AMAZING! Both books are packed with insights and information on the importance of plant based diet from a seriously but readable scientific perspective. *Whole* is easier to read for the layman.

***Over-the-Counter Natural Cures* by Shane Ellison, M.S. The content is sound and this author is "candid" to say the least. He draws on his experience as a pharmaceutical chemist - a profession he found too personally compromising. His Cancer chapter is one of his best (available online free in pdf). He gets a little into "the vernacular", but he is passionate about the truth.

**Water for Health, for Healing, for Life* by Dr. F. Batmanghelidj, M.D. A Fascinating and helpful book. He actually conducted a scientific study using water as his only treatment option while held in an Iranian prison and gave up early release to finish the study.

**The Omega-3 Miracle* by Garry Gordon, M.D., D.O., and Herb Joiner-Bey, N.D. A good deal of information about fatty acids as protection against disease including cancer. A good book to add to Dr. Budwig's books. Includes a helpful index.

**Beta Glucan: Nature's Secret* by Dr. Vaclav Vetvicka, PhD (foremost researcher on the glyco-nutrient, Beta 1.3d Glucan, Dr. Vetvicka is at University of Louisville, KY). This book may be scientifically tedious for some, but there is a website that may simplify main points. www.glucan.us

**Cancer: Natural Cures They Don't Want You to Know About.* by K.A. Thomas. Concise descriptions of a number of protocols often used against cancer symptoms. Compiled information reported by a woman who needed the information for a family member.

**The Acid Alkaline Food Guide: A quick reference to foods & their effect on pH levels* by Brown and Trivieri, Jr. A handy reference book on acid/alkaline balance as related to diet.

Anatomy of an Illness as Perceived by the Patient by Norman Cousins. This is a very interesting book with insights only a personal experience can yield. As a world renowned journalist, Cousins interjects vignettes of what he learned from people like Pablo Casals and Dr. Albert Schweitzer and the lessons are profound and applicable to us today for soul healing.

**Love, Medicine & Miracles* by Bernie S. Siegel, M.D. Dr. Siegel, a surgeon, learned a great deal about what he terms, "self healing", from his "exceptional patients" who refused to let their medical issues kill them. He shares what he learned about their common traits.

***Who Switched Off My Brain? New Edition* by Dr. Caroline Leaf, PhD. Leaf is a Christian psychologist who has a way of teaching complex and important brain mechanisms so that a layman can apply in order to move into wholeness.

The Believer's Authority by Kenneth E. Hagin. A short rich book explaining our spiritual authority in Christ. This book is a classic from a tremendously discerning and anointed minister.

***The Physics of Heaven.* by Judy Franklin and Ellyn Davis. Davis has a background in quantum physics and both women are mature Christians well familiar with Scripture. A number of very insightful people have contributed chapters including Bob Jones, Bill Johnson, David Van Koevering, Ray Hughes, Beni Johnson, Cal Pierce, Dan McCollam, Jonathan Welton, and Larry

Randolph. This is a one of a kind book with very practical spiritual and quantum perspectives.

****Foods to Fight Cancer– Essential Foods to Help Prevent Cancer* by Richard Béliveau, PhD and Denis Gingras, PhD. This book is extremely well presented and I would say a MUST for the library of a person serious about eating to "slam the door on cancer". It is a quick reference book that explains why certain foods fight cancer.

**The Hallelujah Diet by George Malkmus. This book is chocked full of information both Biblical and Scientific as well as personal experience. Malkmus' own testimony is a faith builder. The website www.hacres.org offers much useful instruction.

*** *Fresh Vegetable and Fruit Juices, Diet and Salad, Become Younger.* Three different books by Dr. N. W. Walker, D. Sc. (like a British PhD). Just get the "Juice Book" and do it. He has an amazing testimony. These are ageless books. They encouraged me to "go ahead and make my own fresh vegetable juice".

****Anticancer: A New Way of Life* by David Servan Schreiber, M.D., PhD and healed of cancer himself. This book is extremely helpful. Being an M.D., the writer has difficulty giving up some of his allopathic medicine indoctrination but he eventually does so without saying so. He does good work on "Nutraceuticals"- a word he coined to point out foods that MUST be eaten for health and why. Good index.

****Cancer-Free: Your Guide to Gentle, Non-toxic Healing* (2nd ed) by Bill Henderson
This book got my program "jump started" while I did my own research. I read many of the resources cited in this book. I did not subscribe to everything in the book because it deals with many alternative treatments, but it taught me much.

****Biology of Belief* by Bruce Lipton, PhD. An easy to read and fascinatingly edifying book about biological revelations since Einstein and others' discovery of quantum physics. Lipton puts it all in layman's terms. I consider it a must read for anyone who wants to understand where medicine cannot avoid going and soon. IMPORTANT CELL MEMBRANE INFORMATION WITH EASY ILLUSTRATIONS.

****Molecules of Emotion* by Dr. Candace B. Pert, PhD and pharmacologist. This research scientist discovered important protein receptors on cells that chemically explains the impact of emotions on health and, further, verified the mind-body connection in health.

**Everything You Need to Know to Feel Go(o)d by Dr. Candace B. Pert (see above).

***The Case for Alternative Health Care– Understanding, Surviving, and Thriving in the Midst of Our Collapsing Health Care System by Thomas K. Okler, P.T. This book elaborates upon the "dry (healthy) state" and "wet (disease) state" I discuss and much more. Ockler has been on both sides of the health care industry and has great insight.

The Golden Seven Plus One by Dr. C. Samuel West N.D and chemist. The book that pulled together the rest of my research into sequential descriptions of the conditions that describe health and disease at the cellular (and ultimately may be out of print but I found it "used" on www.amazon.com. A great resource but it takes a lot of time to work through.

*Your Body Believes Every Word You Say by Barbara Levine. She uses her own testimony to illustrate. Good information and easier to follow than some other books on this topic.

** Rethinking Pasteur's Germ Theory by Nancy Appleton (also author of Lick the Sugar Habit). This is an engaging and well-researched book that deals with both individual homeostasis but also the need for changing medical paradigm. There is information in this book about infectious disease that you won't readily find elsewhere (yet).

Rethinking Cancer and Detoxification (two books) by Ruth Sackman. I gleaned MUCH good information from this book and found other resources to check out. It very much stresses alternative "cures". Sackman, who lost her daughter to conventionally treated cancer, founded the Foundation for Alternative Cancer Treatment. www.rethinkingcancer.org

Sick and Tired? Reclaim Your Inner Terrain by Robert O. Young, Ph.D and Shelley R Young. L.M.T. There is a great deal of information about the fallacies within "the germ theory" and much explanation of the power and importance of a healthy inner terrain. It would have been a stronger book had the writers not seemed to try to "explain around God" on some points. They also don't appreciate mushrooms, which most other resources do.

Beating Cancer With Nutrition by Dr. Patrick Quillin. Quillin has a great deal of education and hands on experience.

**Vitamins & Minerals Demystified: A self-teaching guide by Dr. Steve Blake. Clear, concise and helpful with good visual aids.

Websites/Online Articles:
www.internationalwellnessdirectory
There are several well-researched and well-written articles on this site.
"Johanna Budwig Revisited" explains a lot about the important work of
Dr. Budwig and "The Lost History of Medicine" discusses (accurately per
my research) the opposing medical theories of Louis Pasteur and Antoine
BeChamp which explain "modern medicine's" tunnel vision on germs.

Here are some "articles" to "Search Online":
"Cell Biochemistry: Biochemistry of the stress Response" by Eran
Kalmanovich, 2003.

"What is a Healthy Cell?" Greg Ciola interviews Gary Tunsky May 26, 2006.

"Neo Health": A New Paradigm in Essential Health Protocols" by Keith
Armour
MacFarlane A good elaboration on the work of Dr. C. Samuel West.

"The Greatest Health Discovery" by Keith MacFarlane. Lots of good information on the lymphatic system.

"Science of Emotions and Consciousness" by Candace B. Pert, PhD with Nancy
Marriott.

"Healing the Divide: Emerging Perspectives on Mind-Body Unity" by Carrie
Grossman for Douglas Brady.
"Fighting Cancer" Laboratory of Dr. Vaclav Vetvicka, MD. www.glucan.us This
website provides the science for Beta Glucan a well studied immune system
booster.

A Public Domain "Chronological Table of The Miracles of Christ" by David
Brown can be found at: http://www.ccel.org/j/jfb/jfb/JFB00F.htm . It links
to every Scriptural location for each miracle and gives location miracles
occurred. You can just search the title.

YouTube Videos:
My exercise video on YouTube: "Slam the Door on Cancer Exercise Routine"
http://youtu.be/lIWoEaiHEV8

Search YouTube "Tom Ockler Core Breathing Videos" or visit www.
tomocklerpt.com and click on the core breathing videos tab in the list at the bottom of home page.

Masaru Emoto's Water Crystal Photos: This is a beautiful presentation of the crystals of water exposed to words. http://youtu.be/tAvzsjcBtx8

There are numerous YouTube Videos by Charles and Annette Capps dealing with the impact of our words and thoughts as well as Quantum Faith. Just go to www.youtube.com and then search the Capps names.

Video by Glenda Linkous entitled "Power of Words". http://youtu.be/rDx-9dxxRnbO This is a pretty interesting video as well.

Recent message from Heidi Baker, PhD, whose ministry has transformed nations. I believe it speaks to our premise in this book and urge you to take an hour and build up your soul. She is one of a kind. You can search "Heidi Baker Choice 2013 Video" also. http://www.youtube.com/watch?v=PaXZIfa3gpE&feature=share&list=TLDUxV_LXrOjDHq_-bEYmZ84Jm2tOAFNqS .

Healing Room Ministries:
There are healing room ministries worldwide rooted in the ministry of John G. Lake, one of "God's Great Generals". The headquarters is in Spokane, WA, USA with branches in many states and countries. The website is www.healing-rooms.com and the director is Cal Pierce.

Cal Pierce has a presentation entitled "Destroying Cancer" which is available as either CD or mp3 download from the bookstore on the above website. I HIGHLY recommend it.

Bethel Church, Redding, California, USA also has a healing room ministry that people visit from all over the world. www.ibethel.org/healing-rooms-ministry will get you to the information page.

Bethel Church of Redding has a sort of "flock of churches" they work with all over the world. There is a Bethel of Atlanta, GA and a Bethel of Cleveland. Bethel's lead pastor is Bill Johnson (quoted in this book) with his wife, Beni Johnson, a gifted intercessor, health advocate, and author.

www.beinhealth.com is the website of the "For My Life" healing programs led by Rev. Henry W. Wright (quoted in this book) in Thomaston, GA, USA. The website navigates you to programs on their campus and elsewhere.

Podcasts to Feed You Scriptural Encouragement:
Bethel Church, Redding, CA. Sermon of the Week.
http://podcasts.ibethel.org/podcasts.rss

Bethel Atlanta, GA. Sermon of the Week.
http://ibethelatlanta.org/podcast/feed.xml

Kris and Kathy Vallotton, authors and director of Bethel School of
Supernatural Ministry, Bethel Church, Redding, CA.
http://feeds.feedburner.com/kvministries

Pastor Joseph Prince, author of several very encouraging books and sound
teacher of hope. http://feeds.feedburner.com/JosephPrinceAudioPodcast

Frank Viola Podcasts
http://ptmin.podbean.com/feed/

Appendix Three

Food Nutraceuticals

*And God said, See, I have given you every plant yielding seed
that is on the face of all the land and every tree with seed in its fruit;
you shall have them for food.* (Genesis 1:29)

This Appendix charts foods and food groups that contain molecules with
impact on the came bodily mechanisms.

DETOXIFY:
Green Tea (especially Japanese varieties)
Cruciferous Vegetables (Cabbage, Cauliflower, Broccoli, Brussels Sprouts, etc)
Garlic, onions
Mushrooms such as shiitake, maitake, enokidake, cremini, portobello, oyster
(Available in a spice dispenser.)
Sea Vegetables such as NORI, kelp, dulse, kombu, wakame, arame (Available
dried and flaked to use as a table seasoning in lieu of salt.)
Berries: blueberries, strawberries, cranberries, raspberries, blackberries (fresh
or frozen)
Fresh fruits such as apples, plums, peaches, nectarines (organic or peeled)
Oranges, tangerines, lemons
Avocados
Cilantro (fresh) is commonly used in heavy metal detoxification as well as
radiation detox.

INHIBITS INFLAMMATION:
Cruciferous Vegetables (Cabbage, Cauliflower, Broccoli, Brussels Sprouts, etc)
Parsley, Celery
Mushrooms such as shiitake, maitake, enokidake, cremini, portobello, oyster
Garlic, onions
Pomegranate Juice without sugar and pomegranate fruit fresh

Berries: blueberries, strawberries, cranberries, raspberries, blackberries, elder-berries (fresh or frozen)
Avocados
Omega 3 Fatty Acids (walnuts, flax oil, wild caught salmon)

BOOST IMMUNE SYSTEM:
Diet rich in fresh or lightly steamed or stir fried vegetables
Fresh fruits such as apples, plums, peaches, nectarines (organic or peeled)
Garlic, onions
Mushrooms such as shiitake, maitake, enokidake, cremini, portobello, oyster
Avocados
Citrus fruit (not processed juice) with natural pulp

STIMULATES APOPTOSIS (CELL SUICIDE) and/or NATURAL KILLER CELLS:
Cruciferous Vegetables (Cabbage, Cauliflower, Broccoli, Brussels Sprouts, etc)
Soy
Bright colored vegetables and fruits rich in carotenoids like: carrots, yams, squash, pumpkins, tomatoes, persimmons, apricots, beets.
Mushrooms such as shiitake, maitake, enokidake, cremini, portobello, oyster
Sea Vegetables such as NORI, kelp, dulse, kombu, wakame, arame

INHIBITS PROLIFERATION OF TUMOR CELLS:
Cruciferous Vegetables (Cabbage, Broccoli, Brussels Sprouts, etc)
Sea Vegetables such as NORI, kelp, dulse, kombu, wakame, fucoidan,
Garlic, onions, leeks, shallots, chives
Berries: blueberries, strawberries, cranberries, raspberries, blackberries (fresh or frozen)
Flavonoids in all vegetables – especially onions, broccoli, greens
Apples and grapes, grapefruit, figs
Red peppers
Dark Chocolate (more than 70% cocoa) in moderation
Omega 3 Fatty acids (as in walnuts, flax oil, wild caught salmon)
Soy

INHIBITS INVASION OF TUMOR CELLS TO OTHER TISSUE:
Garlic, onions, leeks, shallots, chives
Broccoli (especially sprouts)
Red peppers
Nuts

INHIBITS ANGIOGENESIS (GROWTH OF TUMOR BLOOD SUPPLY):
Green Tea (especially Japanese Varieties) Cruciferous Vegetables (Cabbage, Cauliflower, Broccoli, Brussels Sprouts
Parsley, Celery
Berries: blueberries, strawberries, cranberries, raspberries, blackberries (fresh or frozen)
Grapes
Omega 3 Fatty Acids (Walnuts, Flax oil, wild caught salmon)
Soy
Dark Chocolate (greater than 70% cocoa)
Tomatoes (cooked especially with olive oil on low heat)

I am reporting from two main sources in the above lists: *Anti-Cancer: A New Way of Life*, by Dr. David Servan-Schreiber, M.D., PhD and *Foods to Fight Cancer*, by Richard Béliveau, PhD and Denis Gingras, PhD.

NOTE ABOUT CAROTENOIDS:
Shane Ellison, www.thepeopleschemist.com has a great blog post on "Making his kids eat sunscreen" which is a humorous way of saying his kids eat their vegetables rich in carotenoids like dark green leafy vegetables, carrots, yams, squash. Shane explains that these colorful molecules protect plants and animals from excess sunshine as melanin does.

Points to Remember:
Eating good quality food curbs appetite, nourishes, and prevents disease so that you get more "bang for you food buck" than eating larger volumes of cheaper manufactured foods full of health destroying molecules that do not satisfy hunger.

- ❖ Vegetables and Fruit heal body cells and prevent disease.
- ❖ Avoid smoked and preserved or salted foods such as bacon, sausages, deli meats.
- ❖ AVOID EATING FOODS THAT MAKE YOU THIRSTY.
- ❖ Reduce meat consumption and avoid charred meats cooked over a flame.
- ❖ Eat a variety of foods and be creative.
- ❖ Eat fruit at times other than meals.

- ❖ Eat moderately and regularly and include a lot of food naturally rich in water.
- ❖ Drink plenty of pure filtered or distilled water not from plastic bottles.
- ❖ Eat with pleasure– enjoy good company and think good thoughts while eating.
- ❖ Include smoothies, salads, and sprouts (especially broccoli sprouts) regularly.
- ❖ Drink green tea.
- ❖ EXERCISE– avoid stagnation
- ❖ BREATH WELL
- ❖ Get REAL SUNSHINE regularly
- ❖ Consider your SKIN as "another mouth" and take care what you allow it to absorb.

Appendix Four

Categories of Nutraceutical Spices

This appendix charts of spices is compiled from the work of Dr. Bharat B. Aggarwal, University of Texas M.D. Anderson Cancer Center, as the lead writer of a NIH manuscript entitled: "Molecular Targets of Nutraceuticals Derived from dietary Spices: Potential Role in suppression of Inflammation and Tumorigenesis (tumor growth)".

INHIBITS INFLAMMATION:
Allspice, Anise, Basil, Bay Leaves, Black Pepper, Caraway, Cardamom, Celery Seed, Chives, Cinnamon, Cloves, Cilantro/Coriander Seed, Dill, Fennel, GARLIC, GINGER, Horseradish, Marjoram, Peppermint, MUSTARD, Nutmeg, Onion, Paprika, Parsley, Red Pepper, Rosemary, Sage, Sesame seed, Tarragon, Thyme, TURMERIC (curcumin), White Pepper.

STIMULATES APOPTOSIS (CELL SUICIDE):
Basil, Dill, Fennel, GARLIC, GINGER, Horseradish, Peppermint, Mustard seed, Nutmeg, Paprika, Parsley, Red Pepper, ROSEMARY, Saffron, Sesame Seed, Thyme.

INHIBITS PROLIFERATION (TUMOR CELL GROWTH):
Allspice, Basil, Bay Leaves, Black Pepper, Caraway, Cardamom, Celery Seed, Cinnamon, Cloves, Coriander, Cumin, Dill, Fennel, GARLIC, Horseradish, Mustard, Nutmeg, Onion, Paprika, Parsley, Red Pepper, Rosemary, Saffron, Sage, Sesame Seed, Tamarind, Tarragon, TURMERIC.

INHIBITS INVASION OF TUMOR CELLS INTO OTHER TISSUE:
Allspice, Basil, Bay Leaves, Cardamom, GARLIC, Ginger, Horseradish, Mustard seed, Onion, Oregano, Red Pepper, Saffron, Sesame Seed, Thyme, turmeric, Vanilla.

INHIBITION OF ANGIOGENESIS (GROWTH OF TUMOR BLOOD SUPPLY):
Asafetida, Caraway, Cardamom, Chives, Cilantro/Coriander Seeds, GARLIC, Ginger, Horseradish, Mustard, Oregano, Red Pepper, Sesame Seed, Tarragon, Thyme, TURMERIC

Note: I have emphasized with capitalization and bold face those spices with more than one nutraceutical molecule. Obviously Garlic and some others are particularly potent; however, that doesn't mean others are weak. There may be a particular spice with only one nutraceutical molecule, but it may be a very active one. Eating a variety IS "the spice of life".

Appendix Five

Inflammatory Cascade of Events

The following reveals an illustration of the cascade of events that adds injury to insult of body and soul by degrading the body's "inner terrain", a process that makes the body hospitable to cancer. This "cascade of events" is an illustration and not meant to be a comprehensive overview of every possible cause of cancer.

1. THE PROLONGED "INSULT": Repeated or persistent insult (stress) causes **prolonged** stimulation of certain immune system chemicals. These chemicals are naturally released to temporarily implement tissue healing, fight infection or instigate normal "fight or flight" defense reactions.

2. THE IMMUNE SYSTEM RESPONSE: Immune system chemicals move into the bloodstream making vessel walls more porous so they leak extra fluid (plasma) into the space between cells. Extra blood proteins also pass into that space.

3. FOOD AND OXYGEN SUPPLY INTERRUPTED: The extra fluid and proteins push closely packed body cells apart so that artery capillaries can't efficiently deliver food and oxygen to cells nor can the vein and lymph capillaries pick up the extra fluid, extra proteins and the excreted cellular wastes.

4. ENERGY GENERATION BLOCKED: Energy generation in the cells is hampered because the electrically charged extra blood proteins in the extra fluid between cells interfere with "pumps" in the cell membranes that must constantly move charged particles into and out of the cells generating electrical energy. There are online animations of these "sodium/potassium pumps".

5. LIFE PROCESSES HAMPERED: Thus, "wet or disease state" persists and the body cells start to manifest evidence of being under siege without the necessary energy or supplies to normally eat, breathe, reproduce, excrete, and do their "assigned" jobs for the body.

6. SURVIVAL MODE BEGINS: As the "wet disease state" persists, the cells' terrain continues to deteriorate so that they are essentially "gasping for oxygen". Then, without constantly receiving that oxygen and fresh glucose (food) as well as other necessary minerals, hormones, and essential molecules, cells shift into "survival mode" and do whatever they can to stay alive as long as possible. DNA is damaged.

7. CANCER FRIENDLY ENVIRONMENT: Instead of using oxygen to normally metabolize glucose and generate energy, the cells are forced to plan B by fermenting glucose producing lactic acid waste and pushing the body into abnormal acidity (a state cancer loves and our blood cannot tolerate).

8. BODILY SYMPTOMS ARISE. The body in which these cells live becomes fatigued and is likely in pain from the blocked oxygenation. In short, the body cells are quite unhappy, struggling to survive, and making the person living in that body very uncomfortable.

9. DISEASE TAKES HOLD: Health has been undermined. While the entire body is involved, certain areas or sites may manifest more specific symptoms than others for various reasons.

10. DEATH: The "disease state" is established and, without a reverse back to the "healthy state", disease will be able to continue degrading the "quality of life" for the entire body. Ultimately, death to cells means death to the body but numerous "disease" conditions or "groups of symptoms" can manifest and make death a slow, painful process. The body will fight to live as long as possible, and, as my own story illustrates, we are capable of amazing reversal of the "disease state" back to the "healthy state".

Is the above list over simplified? Somewhat, but it illustrates that **cells become unhealthy for a reason** and cancer is an insidiously perverse counterfeit "survival process" at the cellular level. It can originate at the site of traumatic "insult" or it can manifest organically at a point of weakness or particularly heavy stress. Regardless, it affects the entire body. Disease doesn't "just happen". There is a cause – a "head to cut off the bully" and cancer, indeed disease, is a bully.

("Cascade of Events" is partially extrapolated from Dr. C. Samuel West's work published in his book, *The Golden Seven Plus One*.)

Printed in Great Britain
by Amazon.co.uk, Ltd.,
Marston Gate.